ANATOMY AND PHYSIOLOGY STUDY GUIDE
FOR SPEECH AND HEARING

ANATOMY AND PHYSIOLOGY STUDY GUIDE FOR SPEECH AND HEARING

William R. Culbertson, Ph.D.

Stephanie S. Cotton, M.A.

Dennis C. Tanner, Ph.D.

Northern Arizona University

Flagstaff, Arizona

PLURAL
PUBLISHING
INC.

SAN DIEGO
OXFORD
BRISBANE

5521 Ruffin Road
San Diego, CA 92123

e-mail: info@pluralpublishing.com
Web site: http://www.pluralpublishing.com

49 Bath Street
Abingdon, Oxfordshire OX14 1EA
United Kingdom

Typeset in 12/14 Helvetica by Flanagan's Publishing Services, Inc.
Printed in the United States of America by McNaughton and Gunn

ISBN-13: 978-1-59756-026-9
ISBN-10: 1-59756-026-X
Library of Congress Control Number: 2005908654

Contents

Introduction

The *Anatomy and Physiology Study Guide for Speech and Hearing* is intended to augment a one semester (or two quarters) undergraduate course in anatomy and physiology of human communication. Students should regard this material as only one of several training modalities in this field.

The words "anatomy" and "physiology" often intimidate the entry-level student. Course titles such as these create thoughts of memorizing long lists of Latin words and trying to comprehend vague concepts of bodily sites and functions. These fears are well-founded if the student tries to absorb advanced material from the start. All too often, the result is an elaborate vocabulary built upon a poor foundation, and the student may feel overwhelmed.

The authors intentionally omitted a large amount of information from the content of these units. This was not because the material was unimportant, but because there is only so much material an undergraduate student should be expected to learn and retain at the introductory level. That is, the purpose of this study guide is to help the student develop a starting point from which to search for additional information as the need arises.

There are many fine texts available in anatomy and physiology that contain important material beyond that which is covered in this book. Much or most of it is better advanced to "reference" status. Some additional texts are listed in the reference section.

In addition to the need to simplify the material for the student, there is the matter of time. Most communication sciences programs allow one term for anatomy and physiology courses. Professors may find themselves lecturing rapidly, like radio announcers, to include all the material within the time limits of the term. Limitations on the extent of this study guide resulted from many years of full-time clinical and teaching experience.

The units are designed according to a three-step study sequence. First, the student should become familiar with the stated **objectives**, and check these again at the completion of the unit. Accomplishment of these goals should provide a very well-rounded idea of anatomy and physiology as it generally applies to the practice of speech-language pathology and audiology.

Next, the student should follow the **study outline**. Study outlines map the course of study, and are arranged to help students reach unit goals. They list important concepts, structures, and/or functions, arranged in progressively smaller "chunks," to ease the assimilation of each topic.

These outlines include italicized questions and activities to help the student absorb the material. Space is provided to write the necessary and relevant descriptions, definitions, and/or explanations, but the assiduous student may need additional space in a separate notebook. The information required to complete the outlines may come from many sources, including text(s), specimens, models, slides, videos, and lectures. Instructors, of course, may add or delete topics according to course requirements.

Finally, after the student feels comfortable with the material, she or he should take the **self-tests**, review the answers, and regard the incorrect ones as feedback on the extent to which the unit is completed. The uses of the self-tests are limited by the student's imagination and personal tastes. A student may use these tests as a private means of checking study progress, or use them in groups and share the results. The instructor may employ these tests to allow practice in the class, or to reduce anxiety associated with an actual examination. They are valuable learning experiences.

The illustrations in this study guide accompany the self-tests. Students should fill in the blanks with the names of the structures indicated. Copies of these illustrations with the structures named are included in the section with the answers to the self-tests. The authors wish to acknowledge the patience and hard work of Susan Durning and Erica Fuchs in the preparation of these illustrations.

A solid background in anatomy and physiology can help the aspiring speech language pathologist or audiologist prepare for the profession in a stimulating and productive way. The purpose of this study guide is to help establish that background. If the study of anatomy and physiology can become more enjoyable through use of this text, then the authors' hopes will be realized, as well.

UNIT 1

INTRODUCTION TO ANATOMY AND PHYSIOLOGY

As students begin the study of anatomy and physiology for speech and hearing, they should absorb some general ideas and basic concepts. The ancient study of the forms and functions of the human body is as rooted in culture as it is in science. Terms and concepts about human life vary with language and philosophy.

The approach of this book is based on the *Terminologica Anatomica (TA)*, conceived in 1998 in Paris, France. TA contains terms in both Latin and the equivalent English.

Introduction to anatomy and physiology should start with presentations of the disciplines, including their foci, similarities, and differences. Next, the student should examine specializations within each field to gain appreciation for the breadth of study that is possible.

The introductory section presents guidelines for learning the language of anatomy and physiology in the speech and hearing sciences. Terms apply to **structures** and **locations**, **positions** and **relationships**, **processes**, and **actions**. Mastery of the information contained in the first unit will provide a solid foundation for mastery of material in future units.

The following are the objectives for the unit on the introduction to anatomy and physiology. Success in accomplishing these objectives should prepare the student for further study of the following units. The student can determine mastery of the material presented in Unit 1 by checking the appropriate box as each goal is completed.

✐ ☐ 1. Differentiate between the sciences of anatomy and physiology.

✐ ☐ 2. Describe the following subdivisions of anatomy:
   a. descriptive or systemic anatomy
   b. applied or practical anatomy
   c. microscopic anatomy
   d. developmental anatomy
   e. geriatric anatomy

✐ ☐ 3. Describe the following subdivisions of physiology:
   a. general physiology
   b. applied physiology
   c. experimental physiology
   d. special physiology
   e. pathologic physiology

✐ ☐ 4. Describe the anatomic position with reference to:
   a. the posture of the body
   b. the position of the limbs
   c. the direction of the eyes
   d. the position of the palms

✐ ☐ 5. Given diagrams of the human form from different perspectives, identify the following planes:
   a. median or midsagittal plane
   b. sagittal plane
   c. coronal plane
   d. transverse or horizontal plane

6. After defining the following anatomic terms, use them to describe the location of any structure or to compare the locations of two or more structures:

   a. peripheral/central
   b. ventral/dorsal
   c. anterior/posterior
   d. superficial/deep
   e. superior/inferior
   f. medial/lateral
   g. proximal/distal
   h. caudal/rostral (cranial)
   i. external/internal

I.   Definitions

Fill in the spaces below with the definitions of each science. How do the sciences of anatomy and physiology complement one another?

    A.   Anatomy

    B.   Physiology

II.   Subdivisions of Anatomy

Describe each of the following specialized branches in the science of anatomy. Which branches have the most direct relevance to speech-language pathology and audiology? Explain the relevance.

    A.   Descriptive Anatomy

    B.   Applied Anatomy

    C.   Microscopic Anatomy

    D.   Developmental Anatomy

E.   Geriatric Anatomy

III.   Subdivisions of Physiology

Fill in the spaces with your definitions of the following specialized branches of physiology. Describe how each has relevance to the fields of audiology and speech-language pathology.

A.   General Physiology

B.   Applied Physiology

C.   Experimental Physiology

D.   Special Physiology

E.   Pathologic Physiology

IV.   Anatomic Position

A.   Position

In the space provided below, draw a figure of a person facing you and standing in the anatomic position. Why is it important to have a conventional anatomic position?

1.   Body Standing Erect

2.   Face Forward

3.   Arms Extended Downward at Sides

4.   Palms Forward

B.   Names of Major Topographic Regions

Locate these regions in your drawing.

1.   Cranial Region

2.   Cervical Region

3.   Thoracic Region

4.   Abdominal Region

5.   Upper Extremities

6.   Lower Extremities

V.   Anatomic Planes of Reference

Into which sections do these planes divide the body?

A.   Sagittal

B.   Coronal

C.   Transverse (Horizontal)

VI.   Anatomic Location Terms Presented as Antonym (Opposite) Pairs

In which directions do these terms direct the student? Use each term in a sentence to describe the relationship between two known body parts.

A.   Peripheral:

Central:

B.   Ventral:

Dorsal:

C.   Anterior:

Posterior:

D.   Superficial:

Deep:

E.   Superior:

Inferior:

F.   Medial:

       Lateral:

G.   Proximal:

       Distal:

H.   Caudal:

       Rostral (Cranial):

I.   External:

       Internal:

1. The human form, in the anatomic position, is situated with the body posture _____, the palms _____, the eyes _____, the upper extremities _____.

2. The science that studies the functions of living organisms or their parts is _____.

3. The body is divided into anterior and posterior sections by a _____ plane.

4. The body is divided into superior/inferior sections by a _____ plane.

5. The head is _____ to the shoulder.

6. The heel is _____ to the knee.

7. The brain lies inside the skull. The nose is _____ to the brain.

8. The ear lies on the _____ aspect of the skull.

9. The hand is _____ to the elbow.

10. The science that is concerned with the structure of organisms is called _____.

11. The branch of anatomy that deals with the form of the long-lived individual is called _____.

12. The branch of anatomy that deals with the growth of the organism from a single cell to birth is _____ anatomy.

13. The branch of physiology that deals with the changes brought about by the process of disease is _____ physiology.

14.   Research in speech-language pathology is primarily studied in _____

physiology.

UNIT 2

CYTOLOGY AND HISTOLOGY

Familiarity with the basic components of a system provides a foundation for understanding the larger structure and scope of its functions. For the biological mechanisms of human communication, the study of cells and tissues is a good place to start.

Elements comprise molecules that, in myriad aggregations, comprise the various proteins. These proteins form the components of cells, and serve the cells' essential functions through their chemical reactions. At some point, the basic elemental substrates become alive. The attributes that define life invite the deepest contemplation. Living cells aggregate to form the various **tissues** of which our **organs** are formed. Organs interact and coordinate through **systems** to maintain the complex organism.

The single cell represents the unit constituent of the living body. The human body's genetic code causes proliferation and differentiation of the **zygote**, begun as a single cell product of **gamete** union.

Three basic germ layers appear and become the source for the **four basic tissue types**: **connective**, **epithelial**, **muscle**, and **nervous**. Each type has special properties.

As the **zygote** develops into an **embryo**, and later into a **fetus**, discrete structures become visible. Early in fetal development, small arch-shaped ripples appear in its rostral end. These arches are called **branchial arches**. They form the foundations of most of the structures we associate with the peripheral speech and hearing mechanisms.

The human communication mechanism is efficient at its task partly because it is composed of specialized tissues. Special types of connective and epithelial tissues respond to the vibrations of sound energy and air compression to transmit and receive the signals we call speech. Muscle tissue, by virtue of its contractibility, and nervous tissue, through its enhanced excitability, allows the individual to make sounds with the gases of respiration.

Most books on anatomy and physiology consider the body as divided into convenient sections. This division eases study, but the advanced student will soon learn to appreciate the synergy with which all systems must operate. All **cells**, **tissues**, **organs**, and **systems** interact to form a unity in the healthy individual.

The following are the goals for the unit on basic human cells and tissues. The student can determine mastery of the material presented in this unit by checking the appropriate box as each goal as completed.

✐ ☐   1.   Define and give examples of each of these structural units:
- a.   cell
- b.   tissue
- c.   organ
- d.   system

✐ ☐   2.   List the qualities that describe the property of life.

✐ ☐   3.   Describe the cell in terms of its basic substance and two principal constituents.

✐ ☐   4.   Name and describe the four basic tissue types of the human body

✐ ☐   5.   Name and describe the three functional and three anatomic names for articulations (classifications of joints).

✐ ☐   6.   Describe the three germ layers of the developing embryo and major tissues that derive from each.

✐ ☐   7.   Describe branchial arches and the general functions of their derivative structures.

I.   **General Notes**

Fill in the definitions in the spaces below.

   A.   Definition of Cytology

   B.   Definition of Histology

II. **Cytology**

Fill in the cytologic definitions in the spaces provided.

   A.   Definition of the Cell

   B.   Characteristics of Living Matter

   In your own words, describe these characteristics that distinguish living matter from that which is not living.

      1.   Characteristics of Life in All Organisms

         a.   Growth

         b.   Reproduction

         c.   Metabolism

d. Adaptation or Irritability

2. Characteristics of Life in Some Organisms

Define these characteristics. Under each category provide an example of a living organism that does not exhibit the characteristic.

a. Spontaneous Movement

b. Expression of Consciousness

c. Voluntary Use of Senses

C. General Structure of the Cell

Briefly describe the parts and functions of these fundamental cell components.

1. Protoplasm

2. Cytoplasm

3.   **Nucleus**

4.   **Cell Fluids**

5.   **Cell Shape**

What are some common cell shapes? In the boxes below, draw cells of three different shapes.

III.   **Histology**

Fill in the fundamental histologic definitions in the spaces provided.

A.   **Definition of Tissue**

B.   **Four Basic Tissue Types**

Describe the form and function of the following tissue types. Provide at least one specific example of a structure in the human speech and hearing mechanism made up of each tissue type.

1.   **Connective**

2.   Epithelial

3.   Muscle

4.   Nervous

C. Connective Tissue

In the spaces provided explain and provide details to differentiate between the following components of connective tissues.

1. Characteristics of Connective Tissue

    a. Variability of Intercellular Structure

    b. Variability of Form

2. Functions

    a. Structural Binding

    b. Structural Separation

    c. Fatty Connective Tissue Functions

d.   Fluid Connective Tissue Functions

3.   Types of Connective Tissue

Describe each type of connective tissue. Give examples of each in the human communication mechanism.

a.   Loose Connective Tissue

(1)   Areolar Tissue

(2)   Adipose Tissue

(3)   Reticular Tissue

b.   Dense Connective Tissue

(1)   Tendons

(2)   Ligaments

(3)   Aponeuroses

(4)   Fascia

c.   Skeletal Connective Tissue

(1)   Cartilage

(a)   Types of Cartilage

i)   Hyaline

ii)   Elastic

iii)   Fibrous

(2)   **Bone**

Describe bone in terms of the special nature of its intercellular material. Describe the following types of bones and provide an example of a body structure composed of each bone type.

(a)   **Long Bone**

.

(b)   **Short Bone**

(c)   Flat Bone

(d)   Irregular Bone

(3)   **Articulations of the Skeletal System**

What does the term "articulation" mean in anatomy and physiology? Below are two classification systems for joints. Describe the direction and extent of movement each joint allows. What are the advantages of each type? Give examples of each type of joint in the human communication mechanism.

(a)   **Functional Classification of Joints**

i)   Synarthrodial

ii)   Amphiarthrodial

iii)   Diarthrodial

(b)   **Anatomic Classification of Joints**

Describe the following anatomic joint types. To what functional classification does each correspond?

(i)   **Fibrous**

(ii)   **Cartilaginous**

(iii)   **Synovial**

d.   **Divisions of the Skeletal System**

List the structures that comprise these skeletal divisions.

(1)   **Axial Skeleton**

(2)   **Appendicular Skeleton**

4.   **Fluid Connective Tissue**

What characteristic of the intercellular structure of fluid connective tissue distinguishes it? What are the functions of the two fluid tissues?

a.   **Blood**

b.   **Lymph**

D.   **Epithelial Tissue**

1.   **Characteristics of Epithelial Tissue**

Describe these aspects of epithelial tissue in the spaces provided.

a.   **Intercellular Structure**

      b.   Cellular Arrangement

2.   **Functions of Epithelial Tissue**

Explain in your own words how epithelial tissue performs the following functions.

      a.   Protective

      b.   Absorptive

      c.   Secretory

      d.   Glandular

      e.   Sensory

3.   **Types of Epithelial Tissue**

Describe these types of epithelial tissue. Where might they be found within the mechanism for communication?

a. Proper Epithelium

b. Mesothelium

c. Endothelium

d. Descriptive Terms

Define these terms that classify epithelial tissue.

(1) Cell Shape

(a) Squamous

      (b)   **Columnar**

      (c)   **Pyramidal**

      (d)   **Cuboidal**

(2)   **Layers**

      (a)   **Simple**

      (b)   **Stratified**

E. **Muscle Tissue**

Describe muscle tissue in terms of the following.

1. **Characteristics**

2. **Function**

Describe how muscle tissue functions at these progressively larger contractile units.

a. **Sarcomere**

b. **Myofibril**

c. **Muscle Fiber**

d.   **Muscle Fasciculus**

e.   **Muscle**

3.   **Types of Muscle Tissue**

Differentiate between the following types of muscle tissue. Where is each type of muscle tissue found?

a.   **Smooth**

b.   **Cardiac**

c.   **Striated**

4. **Muscle Feedback**

What is the role of conscious and unconscious muscle feedback in the regulation of muscle function for speech?

5. **Muscle Attachment**

To which end of a muscle do the following terms refer?

a. Origin

b. Insertion

6. **Muscle Function Terminology**

Define the following muscle function terms and demonstrate your understanding by describing the movement of a body part or body parts with respect to the terms.

a. Flexion

b. Extension

c. Adduction

      d.   Abduction

  7.   Names of Muscles

Give examples of muscles named according to the characteristics below.

    a.   Shape

    b.   Function

    c.   Location

F.   Nervous Tissue

Describe the following special features of nervous tissue.

  1.   Characteristics

    a.   Excitability

b.   Conductivity

2.   Functions

a.   Excitatory

b.   Inhibitory

3.   Types of Nervous Tissue

a.   Neurons

Describe the following types of neurons. Give examples of locations at which each may be found in the mechanism for human communication. In the boxes provided, draw stylized representations of each type and label the cell body, axons, and dendrites.

(1)   **Unipolar Neurons**

(2)   **Bipolar Neurons**

(3)   **Multipolar Neurons**

b.   **Neuroglial Cells**

Describe the following neuroglial cells. What are their unique functions?

(1)   **Myelinating Glia (Oligodentrocytes)**

(2)   **Astrocytes**

(3)   **Microglia**

(4)   Neurilemma (Ependymal Cells)

G.   **Tissue Differentiation**

Define each of the following germ layers in the spaces provided. Give examples of organs or structures in the speech or hearing mechanism derived from each.

1.   **Germ Layers**

a.   **Endoderm**

b.   **Mesoderm**

c.   **Ectoderm**

2. **Branchial Arches**

   What is a branchial arch? At which end of the embryo do they appear? List the speech and hearing structures that develop from each arch in the spaces provided.

   a. **First Arch (Mandibular Arch)**

   b. **Second Arch (Hyoid Arch)**

   c. **Third Arch**

   d. **Fourth Arch**

e.   Fifth Arch

f.   Sixth Arch

IV.   **Organs and Systems**

A.   **Definitions**

Define the following in the spaces provided.

1.   **System**

2.   **Organ**

B.   **Review of Systems and Their Interactions**

What are the life sustaining functions of the following systems? Which ones have overlaid communicative functions?

1.   **Respiratory**

2.   **Nervous**

3. Muscular

4. Circulatory

5. Digestive

6. Urinary

7. Endocrine

8. Vascular

9. Skeletal

10. Integumentary

11. Articular

1.   A cell is composed of _____ .

2.   Four characteristics that identify an entity as being alive are:

   a.   _____

   b.   _____

   c.   _____

   d.   _____

3.   The study of collections of cells that have similar structures and functions is called _____ .

4.   The thicker part of the protoplasm of a cell is called the _____ .

5.   Name the tissue types that have the following special characteristics:

   a.   Characterized by irritability _____ .

   b.   Forms a protective sheath covering the interior and exterior surfaces of the body _____ .

   c.   Mediates body movements by virtue of contractile properties _____ .

   d.   Binds the body structures together and aids in body maintenance _____ .

   e.   Conducts changes in electrical potential _____ .

6.   Indicate from which germ layers the following structures are derived:

   a.   The brain _____ .

   b.   The muscles of the tongue _____ .

   c.   The cranial nerves _____ .

    d.   The jaw bone _____.

    e.   The lungs _____.

7.   The branchial skeleton includes the _____ and _____ bones, as well as the _____ and _____ cartilages.

8.   The primary function of the branchial and hypobranchial musculature is

    _____.

9.   Embryonic cells differentiate into three distinct groups called _____.

10.   Joints that move freely are called _____ or _____.

11.   The type of muscle that is under voluntary control is _____.

12.   What comprises a *motor unit*? _____.

13.   The term applied to the attachment of a muscle to a more movable body part is _____.

14.   Define *organ*. _____

SOMATIC CELL

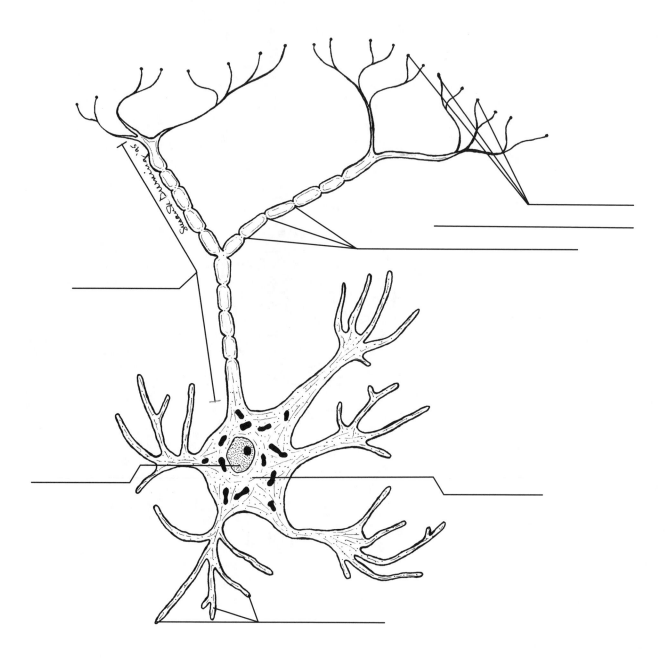

NEURON

UNIT 3

THE RESPIRATORY SYSTEM

The essential function of the respiratory system is to allow the exchange of gases to and from the environment. By virtue of its specialized structure, the respiratory mechanism allows the exchange of **oxygen** from the external atmosphere for **carbon dioxide** from the bloodstream. While the life function of respiration is automatic, human beings have learned to control the respiratory system for the overlaid function of speaking.

The action by which air flows into the lungs is referred to as **inspiration**. Air, and other liquids and gases, flow from higher pressure regions to lower pressure regions. An inward flow of oxygen containing atmospheric air results from contraction of the muscles of inhalation. More than a dozen muscles are involved in this process. Contractions of these muscles increase the size of the thorax vertically, anteroposteriorly, and transversely. As the size of the thorax increases, the pressure inside decreases according to **Boyle's Law**. Certain forces that oppose inspiration must be overcome. They include the small resistance to airflow in the respiratory airway, the resistance to deformation of the respiratory tissue or the elastic recoil of the lungs and thorax, and the fluid pressure of the abdomen.

Expiration is the action by which air flows from the lungs. This flow is caused by a decrease in the dimensions of the thorax and a resulting increase in its internal pressure. Expiratory changes are normally effected by allowing the forces that oppose inspiration to act. At the peak of inspiration, the alveolar pressure is equal to the atmospheric pressure. When the muscles of inspiration relax, the alveolar pressure exceeds that of the atmosphere and causes air to flow out of the lungs. When forceful expulsion of respiratory air is required, the muscles of expiration contract.

The anatomy of the healthy respiratory mechanism creates a dynamic balance among the structures of the torso. The torso, or the body without the head and extremities, is divided into superior and inferior divisions by the dome-shaped **diaphragm**. The diaphragm is also the primary muscle of inhalation. The superior division of the torso, containing the heart, lungs, ribs and muscles, is called the thorax. The inferior division is the **abdomen**. This fluid-filled cavity contains the digestive system and various organs and glands. Function of the muscles of respiration alternately shifts the balance of internal and external pressures between and among the thoracic cavities and the external atmosphere.

Viewing the respiratory system as a **biological pump** is a convenient analogy. This pump compresses the air used for vital functions and for speech purposes. Physiologic terms for respiratory pressures include **alveolar pressure** or pressure within the lungs and **pleural pressure** or pressure within the thorax but outside the lungs. **Abdominal pressure** is the pressure in the abdomen. The volumes or air involved in respiratory functions are measured with a spirometer. **Tidal capacity** is the total volume of air expired during each normal respiratory cycle. **Complemental air** is the maximum volume of air that can be inspired beyond normal inhalation and is also known as **inspiratory reserve**. **Supplemental air**, or **expiratory reserve volume**, is the maximum volume of air that can be expired beyond the end of a normal tidal expiration. **Residual air** volume is the air remaining in the lungs that cannot be exhaled. **Vital capacity** is the total volume of air measurable within the lungs and includes the sum of tidal capacity, complemental air, and supplemental air. Respiratory rates vary with age and activity. Sleep may decrease the rate by as much as 25%.

Respiration for speech is normally a voluntary act, while vegetative breathing is an autonomic function. For speaking, the muscles of the thorax decrease the air pressure inside the lungs at a rate much quicker than that for quiet breathing. This results in a quick inhalation. Then the muscles slowly relax, so the gas inside the lungs will last longer. The speech segment will be longer.

The pressurized gas from the lungs flows upward to power the larynx and create the other sound sources for speech. Without the power provided by the respiratory system, speech would be a series of oral gestures, accompanied by very little sound.

The respiratory pump provides a driving force for the generation of voiced and unvoiced sounds. It provides the energy necessary for a series of valving events that result in the acoustic characteristics of phonemes. Voluntary respiratory behavior plays an important role in the suprasegmental aspects of speech, including loudness, pitch, emphasis, and pauses.

Successful accomplishment of these objectives should give the student a basic understanding of respiratory function in speech production. It should also provide the foundation for the evaluation and treatment of speech disorders. When each objective is accomplished, the student should check the box beside it.

✏️ ☐   1.   Describe two definitions of respiration.

✏️ ☐   2.   Describe the mechanics of physical respiration in terms of the principles of Boyle's law.

✏️ ☐   3.   List the structures and divisions of the upper and lower respiratory tracts.

✏️ ☐   4.   Describe the skeleton of the thorax and abdomen.

✏️ ☐   5.   Describe the mechanics and purposes of respiration for life and for speech.

✏️ ☐   6.   Describe the muscles of inhalation and their functions.

✏️ ☐   7.   Differentiate between the muscles of inhalation and the muscles of exhalation.

✏️ ☐   8.   Describe the following respiratory volumes:

        a.   tidal volume   d.   expiratory reserve.

        b.   vital capacity   e.   residual volume

        c.   inspiratory reserve

✏️ ☐   9.   Describe the different respiratory patterns, including:

        a.   diaphragmatic/abdominal   d.   Cheyne-Stokes

        b.   thoracic   e.   neurogenic hyperventilation

        c.   clavicular   f.   Kussmaul respiration

✏️ ☐ 10.   Describe chronic diseases of the respiratory tract, including asthma, emphysema, chronic bronchitis, and chronic obstructive pulmonary disease (COPD).

I. Two Definitions for Respiration

Fill in the definitions in the spaces provided. Why do we describe respiration in two ways? Why is knowledge of the respiratory system important to speech-language pathologists?

A. Physical

1. Biological Functions

2. Speech Function

B. Chemical

Write the chemical equation for respiration.

II. Structures of the Respiratory Tract

A. Location of the Respiratory System

Describe the general location of the structures for breathing. Which ones are located in the upper part?

1.   Upper Respiratory Tract

2.   Lower Respiratory Tract

B.   Skeleton of the Respiratory Tract

Describe the location of the following structures and indicate how many of each are in the body.

1.   Spinal Column

a.   Vertebrae

(1)   **Structure**

Describe the general structure of a vertebra.

(2)   **Types of Vertebrae**

To which vertebrae do these names refer? How many of each are there?

(a)   **Cervical**

i)   **Special Names for Cervical Vertebrae**

Describe the location of each of these vertebrae.

a)   Atlas

b)   Axis

c)   Vertebra Prominens

(b)   Thoracic

(c)   Lumbar

(d)   Sacral

(e)   Coccygeal

2. Pelvic Girdle

What is the role of the pelvic girdle in respiration?

3. Rib Cage

a. Ribs

b. Sternum

4. Clavicles

5. Scapulae

C. Nose and Nasal Cavity

1. Nares

2. Septum

3. Root

4. Choanae

D. Pharynx

Differentiate between these subdivisions of the pharynx.

1. Nasopharynx

2. Oropharynx

3. Laryngopharynx

E.   Oral Cavity Structure and Function

Describe the locations of these oral landmarks.

1.   Fauces

2.   Triangular Fossa

3.   Tonsils

F.   Laryngopharynx

What is the respiratory function of the larynx?

G.   Trachea

Describe the structure and location of the trachea. What is its location relative to the esophagus?

H.   Bronchial Tree

Differentiate between the following components of the bronchial tree by their location in relation to one another.

     1.   Main Stem Bronchi

     2.   Secondary Bronchi

     3.   Tertiary Bronchi

     4.   Bronchioles

I. **Lungs**

Describe the following structures and characteristics of the lungs in the spaces provided.

1. **Right and Left Lung Differences**

2. **Alveoli**

3. **Pleurae**

   a. **Intrapleural Fluid**

   b. **Visceral Pleura**

   c. **Parietal Pleura**

III. **Mechanics of Respiration**

How does Boyle's law relate to breathing? Demonstrate your understanding by providing an example of Boyle's law at work in something other than respiration.

A.   Boyle's Law

B.   Inspiration and Expiration

    1.   Respiratory Cycle

Define a respiratory cycle. What is the normal I-Fraction (ratio of the duration of inhalation to the duration of the entire cycle) for quiet breathing? Describe the differences between the respiratory cycle for speech and that for quiet breathing.

      a.   Vegetative Breathing.

      b.   Respiration for Speech

2.   **Respiratory Rates**

What are normal rates for an adult, child, and infant? How are these rates measured?

      a.   Adult Respiratory Rate Range

      b.   Child Respiratory Rate Range

      c.   Infant Respiratory Rate Range

3.   **Respiratory Patterns**

Describe the most commonly encountered patterns of respiration? How does the diagnostician identify one? Is there one pattern that is more efficient?

a.   Normal Patterns of Respiration

  (1)   Diaphragmatic/Abdominal

  (2)   Thoracic

  (3)   Clavicular

b.   Pathologic Patterns of Respiration

  Describe these pathologic patterns of respiration.

  (1)   Cheyne-Stokes Respiration

  (2)   Neurogenic Hyperventilation

  (3)   Kussmaul Respiration

C.   Muscles of Respiration

    1.   Function of the Muscles of Respiration

    How do the following movements bring about changes in thoracic volumes?

    a.   Diaphragmatic Movement

    b.   Costal Movement

    (1)   "Pump Handle"

    (2)   "Bucket Handle"

    2.   Inhalation: Active Movement

    a.   Primary Muscles of Inhalation

    Describe the origins and insertions of these muscles.

(1)   Diaphragm

(2)   External Intercostals

b.   Secondary Muscles of Inhalation

Under what conditions will an individual employ these muscles? Describe their origins and insertions.

(1)   Pectoralis Majorus/Minoris

    (2)   Costal Levators

            (a)   12 paired

            (b)   C–7 to T–11

    (3)   Serratus Anteriorus

    (4)   Serratus Posterior Superiorus

    (5)   Latissimus Dorsi

    (6)   Scalenus

            (a)   C-3 through C-6

            (b)   To Ribs 1 & 2

3.   Exhalation

Describe the different manners in which gas is expelled from the respiratory system.

a.   **Passive Movement**

b.   **Active Movement**

(1)   **Muscles of Exhalation**

What is the role of the muscles of expiration in the production of speech?

(a)   **Primary Muscles of Expiration**

Describe the origins and insertions of these muscles.

i)   **Internal Intercostals**

ii)   **Rectus Abdominus**

iii)   **Transversus Abdominus**

iv)   **External Obliques**

v)   **Internal Obliques**

(b)   **Secondary Muscles of Expiration**

Describe the origins and insertions of the secondary muscles of exhalation. Under what circumstances might they be employed?

i)   **Serratus Posterior Inferiorus**

ii)   Quadratus Lumborum

iii)   Subcostals

iv)   Latissimus Dorsi

IV.   Measurement of Respiratory Function

What are the implications of respiratory function testing in the evaluation and treatment of communicative disorders?

A.   Spirometry

Describe the spirometer. Can a speech-language pathologist estimate respiratory efficiency for speech without instrumentation? If so, how?

B.   Volumes

Define the following respiratory volumes. What are normal values?

1.   Vital Capacity

2.   Tidal Volume

3.   Inspiratory Reserve (Complementary)

4.   Expiratory Reserve (Supplementary)

5.   Residual

V.   Diseases of the Respiratory System

Describe these common chronic diseases of respiration. What limitations might be imposed on the effects of speech therapy for individuals suffering from these conditions?

A.   Chronic Obstructive Pulmonary Disease (COPD)

B.   Asthma

C.   **Emphysema**

D.   **Chronic Bronchitis**

1.   What are the two points of view from which we can describe respiration?

     _____ and _____.

2.   Air moves in and out of the respiratory tract coincident with changes in the

     _____ of the thorax in a manner consistent with which law of physics?

     _____.

3.   Identify the following anatomic structures as belonging to either the *upper* or

     lower respiratory tract.

     a. Nasopharynx _____   f. Bronchi   _____

     b. Lungs   _____   g. Pleurae   _____

     c. Oral Cavity   _____   h. Nostrils   _____

     d. Fauces   _____   I. Trachea   _____

     e. Choanae   _____   j. Oropharynx   _____

4.   The *nonbiological* function of respiration is _____.

5.   The respiratory system consists of _____.

6.   A respiratory cycle consists of _____.

7.   The normal respiratory rate for adults is _____.

8.   The operation of Boyle's law is ensured by action of _____.

9.   The primary muscles of inhalation are _____.

10. During normal exhalation, the muscles of respiration _____.

11. The first seven vertebrae are called _____.

12. The lateral movement of ribs 7 to 10 is referred to as _____.

13. The muscles of exhalation contract for _____

    _____.

14. The true ribs attach anteriorly to the _____.

15. A device that measures respiratory volumes is called a _____.

16. The vertebrae closest to the lungs are called _____.

17. The volume of air inhaled and exhaled during any single expiratory cycle is

    called the _____.

18. The quantity of air that can be exhaled after as deep an inhalation as possible

    is called _____.

19. The I-Fraction for speech is approximately _____.

20. Expiratory reserve is also known as _____, and is the term used to

    describe the volume of air that _____.

21. The two *normal* patterns of respiration are called _____.

22. Describe Cheyne-Stokes respiration _____

    _____.

23. What are the rehabilitation implications of COPD? _____.

LEFT LUNG

RIGHT LUNG

THORACIC SKELETON

UNIT 4

THE PHONATORY MECHANISM

The production of speech depends on the transmission of sound waves. One of the main anatomic locations for sound production is the **larynx**. The larynx functions as a valve. Because both food traveling to the stomach and air passing to the lungs begin in the same cavity, the larynx serves a dual purpose. It permits the passage of air to and from the lungs while being capable of closing during swallowing to protect the lungs from food and other foreign bodies. Other functions of the larynx include stabilization of the thorax for body exertions and regulation of airflow in and out of the lungs. The opening at the level of the vocal folds is called the **glottis**. **Phonation** refers to any type of vibratory sound produced at the level of the larynx. Whisper is also a function of partially contracting the vocal folds.

The larynx consists of nine **cartilages**, three of which are paired. The largest is the **thyroid cartilage**. The **cricoid cartilage** resembles a signet ring. The **epiglottis**, which is not vital to humans, snaps down like a trap to help protect the airways during swallowing. The **arytenoids**, **corniculates**, and **cuneiforms** are the paired cartilages.

The cartilages of the larynx are tied to one another by **intrinsic ligaments**. **Extrinsic ligaments** connect the laryngeal cartilages above to the hyoid bone and below to the first tracheal ring. In addition to their functions as connecting tissues, the intrinsic laryngeal ligaments spread thin in some places to form membranes. These membranes play a role in producing the vibrations associated with the voice.

The musculature of the phonatory mechanism moves its structure to adjust its openings and postures. **Intrinsic laryngeal muscles** have both origin and insertion within the laryngeal structure. They are primary to pitch and loudness control. The posterior cricoarytenoid is the only muscle responsible for opening, or abducting, the vocal folds. Adductors are intrinsic muscles responsible for forcefully closing the vocal folds. Tensors and relaxers work to elongate and shorten the vocal folds. **Extrinsic laryngeal muscles** have one connection outside the larynx and are frequently referred to as either suprahyoid or infrahyoid. Suprahyoid muscles help elevate the larynx while infrahyoids (neck strap muscles) are involved in lowering it.

The larynx comprises a portion of the pharynx. This portion is called the **laryngopharynx**. It is divided into three cavities. At the superior end is the vestibular portion. This is the entrance to the airway where the larynx and pharynx divide. The middle division of the laryngopharynx is the ventricle. It is bordered by two sets of tissue folds: the **ventricular (false) vocal folds** at the superior end and the **(true) vocal folds** at the inferior end. Inferior to the ventricle just below the true vocal folds is the **subglottic area** of the laryngopharynx.

The act of producing voiced speech is dependent on respiratory support. The vocal folds rapidly vibrate as the compressed respiratory air travels over their surfaces. The vocal folds are capable of closing rapidly due to both **myoelastic** properties of the laryngeal tissue and Bernoulli's **aerodynamic** principle. Pitch and loudness are a result of fine regulation and coordination between subglottic air pressure and muscle resistance. During elevation of pitch, the mass per unit length of the vocal folds is decreased. Lowering of the pitch is a result of an increase of mass per unit length of the vocal folds. To effect these mass changes, the vocalis muscle and the vocal ligament are adjusted by fine movements of the arytenoid cartilages, which are capable of sliding and rotating in response to intrinsic muscle tension and length.

Mastery of the following objectives should give the student a basic understanding of the form and function of the mechanism we use to produce the voice. Such an understanding will give the student a point of departure for study of the evaluation and treatment of phonatory disorders. Students should check the boxes by the objectives as they accomplish them.

1. Describe the larynx in terms of its physical appearance, location, and functions.

2. Describe the general process of phonation and the glottic cycle.

3. Describe glottal postures and their effects on phonatory source characteristics.

4. Name and identify the major cartilages of the larynx.

5. Describe the articulations of the major laryngeal cartilages.

6. Name and identify the major ligaments and membranes of the larynx.

7. Name and identify the intrinsic muscles of the larynx.

8. Name and identify the three sections of the cavity of the larynx.

9. Differentiate the functions of the intrinsic versus the extrinsic muscles of the larynx.

I.   General Structure and Function

    A.   General Description and Location

        Describe the larynx and its general location.

    B.   Evolution

        What is the function of the larynx in lower animals?

    C.   Biological Function

        Apart from phonation, what are the functions of the laryngeal valve?

D.   **Speech Function**

What is the speech function of the larynx? How does it accomplish this function?

1.   **The Glottis and Vocal Folds**

What is the glottis? Differentiate between abduction and adduction of the vocal folds.

a.   **Abduction**

b.   **Adduction**

2.   Physiology of Normal Phonation

a.   The Glottic Cycle

Describe the following phases of the glottic cycle. Draw a graph of the glottic cycle including percentages of time in each phase to demonstrate your understanding.

(1)   Closed Phase

(2)   Opening Phase

(3)   Closing Phase

(4) **Forces**

Describe the forces at work during the glottic cycle.

(a) **Myoelastic**

(b) **Aerodynamic**

b. **Glottal Frequency**

What are the effects of changes in glottal frequency?

(1) **Average Glottal Frequency**

(a) **Males**

(b) **Females**

(2) **Mechanism for Changing Glottal Frequency**

How do the vocal folds change as pitch increases? How are these changes brought about (i.e., what muscles are responsible for altering pitch)?

c. Glottal Cycle Amplitude

Describe the changes that occur in the glottal cycle as the voice becomes louder.

II. The Framework of the Larynx:

A. The Hyoid Bone

Is the hyoid bone part of the larynx?

1. Structure

a. Corpus

b.   Greater Cornua

c.   Lesser Cornua

2.   Function of the Hyoid Bone

a.   Attachments

b.   Relationship to Tongue and to Larynx

B.   Cartilages of the Larynx

What types of cartilages form the skeleton of the larynx?

1.   Unpaired Cartilages of the Larynx

a. **Thyroid Cartilage**

Describe the thyroid cartilage. What is its size and location in relation to the other laryngeal cartilages?

(1) **Structure**

(a) **Laminae**

Describe the angle of fusion of the thyroid laminae. How does this angle change as the individual develops? Is there any relationship between this angle and the sound of the voice?

(b)   Cornua

b.   Cricoid Cartilage

What are the superior and inferior attachments of the cricoid cartilage?

(1)   Attachments

(2)   Structure

Describe and be able to identify the following parts of the cricoid cartilage.

(a)   Lamina

(b)   Arch

(c)   Articular Surface

c.   Epiglottis

Describe the following structures in the spaces below.

(1)   Structure and Location

(2)   Attachments of the Epiglottis

(3)   Glossoepiglottic Folds

(a)   Epiglottic Valleculae

(b)   Laryngeal Inlet

(4)   Epiglottitis

Why is epiglottitis a life-threatening condition?

2.   Paired Cartilages of the Larynx

a.   Arytenoid Cartilages

Describe the following aspects of the arytenoid cartilages.

(1)   Structure

(a)   Vocal processes

(b)   Muscular processes

(2)   Function

Describe the cricoarytenoid joint. What type of joint is it?

(a)   Movement

Describe the following movements of the arytenoid cartilages.

i)   Abduction/Adduction

ii)   Rotation

iii)   Gliding or Sliding

iv)   Tilting

(b)   **Cartilaginous Glottis**

How much of the glottis is bordered by tissue with underlying cartilage? What are the physiological implications of this fact?

(c)   **Membranous Glottis**

b.　　Minor Paired Cartilages of the Larynx

Describe the locations of these minor cartilages.

(1)　　Corniculate cartilages

(2)　　Cuneiform cartilages

(3)　　Triticeal cartilages

C.　Ligaments of the Larynx

Describe the attachments of each of these ligaments. What are their functions? What differentiates an intrinsic ligament from an extrinsic ligament?

1.　Extrinsic Ligaments

a.   **Thyrohyoid Ligament**

b.   **Cricotracheal Ligament**

2.   **Intrinsic Ligaments**

a. **Conus Elasticus (Cricovocal Membrane)**

(1) **Vocal Ligament**

Describe the Vocal Ligament. What are its anterior and posterior attachments? How does it relate to the cricovocal membrane?

(2) **Cricothyroid Ligament**

Why is the cricothyroid ligament called the most important intrinsic ligament?

b.   Vestibular Ligament

III.   Articulations of the Larynx

A.   Cricothyroid Articulation

Describe the articulation of the thyroid cartilage with the cricoid cartilage.

1.   Rotation About the Horizontal Axis

2.   Gliding

3.   Effect on the Voice

B.   Cricoarytenoid Articulation

Review cricoarytenoid articulation.

1.   Rotation

2.   Gliding or Sliding (Anterior/Posterior and Lateral/Medial)

3.   Tilting

IV.   Cavities of the Larynx (Laryngopharynx)

Describe these divisions of the laryngopharynx in relationship to one another.

A.   Vestibular (Superior) Division

1.   Extends from Inlet to Ventricular Folds

2.   Epiglottis

3.   Aryepiglottic Folds

Draw a diagram representing the cross-section of the laryngeal cavity in the box on the right.

B.   Ventricular (Middle Division)

1.   From Ventricular (Vestibular) Folds to Vocal Folds

2.   Ventricular Folds

Is it possible to adduct the ventricular folds?

a.   Composition

b. Attachments

3. Vocal Folds

Describe these aspects of the vocal folds. Why are these folds called the true vocal folds?

a. Composition

(1) Thyroarytenoid Muscles

(2)   Vocalis Muscles

(3)   Vocal Ligaments

b.   Attachments and Positioning of the Vocal Folds

c.   Glottis

Draw a diagram of the glottis as seen from above. Show which part is intercartilaginous.

(1) **Intermembranous**

(2) **Intercartilaginous**

C. **Infraglottic (Subglottic) Division**

What is the relationship of subglottic air pressure to voice loudness?

V.   Muscles of the Larynx: Intrinsic and Extrinsic

A.   Intrinsic Muscles of the Larynx

Why are these muscles referred to as intrinsic? What is the general function of the intrinsic muscles of the larynx? Describe the origins/insertions and functions of these muscles in the spaces provided.

1.   Muscles That Control Tension/Length of the Vocal Ligament

a.   Cricothyroid

b.   Thyroarytenoid

c. Vocalis

2. Muscles That Control Glottal Aperture

a. Posterior Cricoarytenoid

b. Lateral Cricoarytenoid

c.   Transverse Arytenoid

d.   Oblique Arytenoid

3.   Muscles That Modify Laryngeal Inlet

a.   Aryepiglottic

b.   Thyroepiglottic

c.   Ventricular

B.   **Extrinsic Muscles of the Larynx**

Why are these muscles described as extrinsic? How would you describe the general function of the extrinsic muscles of the larynx? Describe the origins/insertions and the functions of the extrinsic muscles in the spaces provided.

1. **Suprahyoid Muscles**

   a. **Digastric**

   b. **Stylohyoid**

   c. **Mylohyoid**

    d.   Geniohyoid

    e.   Hyoglossus

2.   Infrahyoid

    a.   Sternohyoid

    b.   Omohyoid

    c.   Thyrohyoid

    d.   Sternothyroid

3.   Indirect Displacers of the Larynx

    a.   Palatopharyngeus

    b.   Stylopharyngeus

    c.   Inferior Pharyngeal Constrictor

1. What is the most important biological function of the larynx?

    _____.

2. The trachea is (posterior/anterior) to the esophagus.

3. What is the secondary or overlaid function of the larynx?

    _____.

4. Describe the voice in physiological terms. _____.

5. The perceived pitch of the voice is related to _____.

6. The perceived loudness of the voice is related to what physiologic phenomenon?

    _____.

7. Describe the glottis. _____.

8. The hyoid bone is classified as a part of the _____.

9. The largest cartilage of the larynx is the _____.

10. The lowest cartilage of the larynx is the _____.

11. The flat parts of the thyroid and cricoid cartilages are called the _____.

12. The laryngeal prominence marks location of the _____.

13. The cartilage that is shaped like a signet ring is the _____.

14. The vocal ligaments are attached posteriorly to what structures? _____.

15. Movement of the vocal folds away from the midline is called _____.

16.   The muscles that tense and lengthen the vocal ligaments are the

    a.   posterior arytenoid muscles.

    b.   suprahyoid muscles.

    c.   transverse arytenoid and oblique arytenoid muscles.

    d.   cricothyroid, thyroarytenoid, and vocalis muscles.

17.   Which of the following muscles do not adduct the vocal folds?

    a.   posterior cricoarytenoid muscles.

    b.   lateral cricoarytenoid muscles.

    c.   oblique arytenoid muscles.

    d.   transverse arytenoid muscles.

18.   The lateral and posterior cricoarytenoid muscles attach to the arytenoid cartilages at which structures? _____.

19.   During heavy breathing, what position do the vocal folds assume?

    _____.

20.   Of what kind of joint is the cricoarytenoid joint an example? _____.

21.   The upper free border of the cricothyroid membrane is called the _____.

22.   What distinguishes the intrinsic muscles of the larynx from the extrinsic muscles?

    _____.

23.   Which muscle pair abducts the vocal ligaments? _____.

24.   What are the main functions of the extrinsic muscles of the larynx?

    _____.

25.   What term is used to describe the air pressure inferior to the adducted vocal folds? _____.

26.   What is the average glottal frequency in adult females? _____.

27.   Describe the forces that, according to currently held theories, act to close the

glottis during phonation. _____

_____

_____.

28.   Which muscles make up the vocal folds? _____ and _____.

29.   In which direction does the thyroid cartilage move during deglutition

(swallowing)? _____.

30.   What role do the valleculae play in nomal and disordered swallowing?

_____

_____.

PHONATORY SYSTEM

SKELETON OF THE LARYNX

LATERAL VIEW

POSTERIOR VIEW

LARNYX

ANTERIOR VIEW

UNIT 5

THE ARTICULATORY MECHANISM

The primary functions of the articulatory structures are **mastication** (chewing), **deglutition** (swallowing), and **adjustment** of the opening of the airway. The overlaid function of speech production is the result of millions of years of evolution. Human beings discovered that the extreme flexibility of their **branchial** musculature enabled them to produce a broad array of sounds when they moved in relationship to the less mobile structures of the upper airway.

To produce speech, voiced or unvoiced, the compressed airstream from the lungs is shaped by the muscles and structures of articulation. Sounds produced this way are called **egressive**. Some languages employ sounds created by reversing the flow of air, filling the lungs during speech, with the resulting sounds termed **ingressive**.

Speech is articulated through alteration of the shape of the **vocal tract**. The vocal tract is essentially a tube. It extends from the **glottis** to the openings of the nose and mouth. The structures that are used to alter vocal tract shape are referred to collectively as **articulators**.

Typically, the articulators are divided into fixed and mobile structures. The mobile structures move in relationship to the fixed ones, restricting air or altering the resonating characteristics of the tube of the vocal tract.

The **fixed articulators** are the **upper incisors**, (superior) **alveolar ridge**, and the **hard palate**. The **upper incisors**, in combination with the tongue or lower lip, serve to create high-frequency consonants. The **hard palate**, formed by the maxillae and the palatine bones, separates the nasal and oral cavities. The anterior portion of the hard palate, from which the upper incisors erupt, is the **superior alveolar ridge**. This portion of the maxilla is so important to speech that it is usually considered a separate articulator. Because the inferior alveolar ridge is not used for standard speech articulation, the anatomical locator term is usually dropped. The fixed articulators provide a surface against which to juxtapose the tongue or lips for the alteration of resonance and the modification of airflow.

The mobile articulators are the **lips, mandible, velum, tongue, pharyngeal walls**, and **larynx**. The **lips** form a sphincter at the oral opening. They can occlude the oral cavity, articulate with the teeth, or form a ring through selective contraction of the **orbicularis oris** muscle. The formation of a labial ring serves as a fricative source or changes the resonance of the tract by extending its length and circular dimension. The **mandible** is mobile and adjusts oral cavity opening by elevating and depressing. It works synergistically with the **tongue** to produce the fine adjustments necessary for vowel productions. The tongue is the most important structure of speech articulation. It is a flexible muscular structure covered with mucous membrane. Tongue muscles are divided into **extrinsic** and **intrinsic** groups. Extrinsic muscles have one connection outside the tongue and another within the tongue. Intrinsic muscles have both origin and attachment within the tongue. They are primarily involved in shaping the tongue for movement of food and liquid. They also play an important role making the fine adjustments necessary for vowel and consonant productions. The velum extends posteriorly from the hard palate and is continuous with it. It is a movable structure that serves to couple or uncouple the nasal cavity with the rest of the vocal tract. It is closed during sucking and most speech sound articulation.

The structures and muscles of articulation produce the vowels and consonants of language phonology. These may be described by the amount or **manner** and location or **place** of maximum vocal tract constriction associated with their formations. A third descriptor is the presence or absence of **voicing**. Although all vowels are voiced, some consonants are not. Dynamic patterns of articulator movement, opening and closing the vocal tract in various manners and at various locations, produce the audible **syllables** of speech. The study of speech sounds is **phonetics**. Speech sounds may either form the nuclei of syllables or syllable boundaries.

Accomplishment of the objectives of this unit should provide the student with a basis for understanding the structure and function of the orofacial mechanism and the oropharynx. Checking the boxes beside each goal will help the student mark progress toward that understanding.

✎ ☐ 1. Describe the general anatomy of the vocal tract.

✎ ☐ 2. Describe the functions of the structures of the vocal tract in speech and swallowing.

✎ ☐ 3. Name the bones of the skull.

✎ ☐ 4. Describe the major divisions of the bones of the skull.

✎ ☐ 5. Name the structures of speech articulation.

✎ ☐ 6. Differentiate between the fixed and the mobile speech articulators.

✎ ☐ 7. Identify the cavities of the vocal tract and name the structures in each that are essential to normal speech and swallowing.

✎ ☐ 8. Name the muscles of facial expression essential to speech articulation.

✎ ☐ 9. Name the oral and pharyngeal muscles essential to normal speech and swallowing.

✎ ☐ 10. Describe, in general, the changes associated with normal growth of the head.

✎ ☐ 11. Describe the stages of deglutition.

I.   General Structure and Function of the Vocal Tract

    A.   Structure

        Briefly describe the locations of the following structures of the articulatory mechanism.

        1.   Oral Cavity

            a.   Tongue

            b.   Dental Arches

            c.   Hard Palate

d.   Velum (Soft Palate)

2.   Nasal Cavity

a.   Nares

b.   Choanae

c.   Septum

3.   Pharyngeal Cavity

   a.   Laryngopharynx

   b.   Oropharynx

   c.   Nasopharynx

II.   Function

Describe these functional aspects of the articulatory mechanism as they apply to speech and/or deglutition.

A.   Plosive and Fricative Sources for Obstruent Consonants

How do the structures of the oral cavity function to create constrictions for these sources? Are all obstruent consonants formed by constriction in the oral cavity?

B.   Analogy to Band-Pass Filter for Vowels and Semivowels

Provide an example of how the muscles of the articulatory mechanism modify the phonatory source.

C. General Function

Describe the oral cavity as the entrance to the alimentary canal. Differentiate between the routes of passage and list the structures involved in transferring food to the stomach and air to the lungs.

III. The Skull in General

Describe these structures in the spaces provided.

A. Gross Structure

1. Skull

a. Cranium

(1) Facial Skeleton

(2) Calvaria

b.   Mandible

c.   Hyoid bone

2.   **Cavities of the Cranium**

Describe the locations and contents of these cavities of the cranium.

a.   Cranial Cavity

b.   Orbits

c.   Nasal Cavity

B.   Bone Type

C.   Mechanical Stresses

IV.   Superior Aspect of the Cranium

A.   Calvaria

What portion of the skull comprises the calvaria? Describe the locations of the following bones of the calvaria.

1.   Frontal Bone

2.   Temporal and Sphenoid Bones

3.   Parietal Bones

4.   Occipital Bone

B.   Sutures

What type of joint is a suture? How do these joints change as the individual develops? Describe the locations of the following sutures.

1.   Sagittal

2.   Coronal

3.   Lambdoidal

4.   Pterion (squamosal)

V.   Inferior Aspect of the Cranium

Describe the forms and locations of the following structures in the spaces provided.

A.   Anterior Section

1. **Hard Palate**

    Describe the functions of the hard palate in speech and in deglutition.

    a. **Maxilla**

        (1) **Superior Alveolar Process**

        (2) **Incisive Fossa**

    b. **Palatine Bone**

c.   **Superior Teeth**

Identify the following teeth. Which teeth are essential for articulation of dental phonemes? Draw and label the superior dental arch of an adult in the box below.

(1)   **Incisors**

(a)   **Central**

(b)   **Lateral**

(2)   **Cuspids**

(3)   **Bicuspids**

(4)   **Molars**

2.   **Growth and Development of Teeth**

By what age should the teeth necessary for the articulation of dental consonants erupt?

a. **Teeth Eruption**

Give the normal ages of eruption of the superior dentition.

b. **Anomalies of Occlusion**

Define the following terms for dental occlusion anomalies.

(1) **Axiversion**

(a) **Distoversion**

(b) **Mesioversion**

(2) **Infraversion**

(3) **Supraversion**

(4) **Torsiversion**

B. **Middle Section of the Skull**

Describe the sphenoid and occipital bones as structures of the middle, inferior aspect of the skull.

1. **Nasopharynx**

    Locate the nasopharynx with respect to the inferior aspect of the skull.

2. **Sphenoid Bone**

    a. **Pterygoid Plates**

        Describe the pterygoid plates of the sphenoid bone as points of attachment for pharyngeal muscles.

        (1) **Pterygoid muscles**

            Describe the mandibular movement associated with these muscles. Why is this movement important in mastication?

(2) **Tensor Veli Palatini**

Describe the origins and insertions of this muscle. What role does it play in speech? Describe the hamular processes of the sphenoid bone.

(3) **Levator Veli Palatini**

Describe the origins and insertions of this muscle. What role does it play in speech?

3. **Occipital Bone**

What portion of the occipital bone contributes to speech articulation?

C.   Posterior Section of the Inferior Skull

   1.   Occipital Bone

      Describe the form and function of the following landmarks of the occipital bone in the spaces provided.

      a.   Foramen Magnum

      b.   Occipital Condyles

      c.   Hypoglossal Canals

   2.   Temporal Bones

      Describe the forms and functions of these landmarks of the temporal bones in the spaces provided.

      a.   Squamous Portions

      b.   Petrous Portions

(1) **Auditory Meatuses**

(2) **Bony Labyrinths**

c. **Mastoid Processes**

What muscles attach bilaterally to the sternum, clavicle, and the mastoid process?

d. **Styloid Processes**

What muscles attach to the styloid processes bilaterally?

e.   Jugular Foramina

   (1)   Internal Jugular Veins

   (2)   Glossopharyngeal Nerves

   (3)   Vagus Nerves

   (4)   Accessory Nerves

f.   Carotid Canals

   (1)   Internal Carotid Arteries

(2)   Sympathetic Plexuses

VI.   Anterior Aspect of the Skull

Describe the forms and functions of the structures of the anterior skull in the spaces provided.

A.   The Face

1.   Importance in Communication

a.   Speech

Which facial structures are involved in speech?

b.   Facial Expression

Of what importance is facial expression in communication?

2.   Bones of the Face

Describe the locations of these bones of the face.

a.   Frontal Bone

b.   Maxillae

c.   Zygomatic Bones

d.   Nasal Bones

3.   Landmarks of the Face

Write the locations of these facial landmarks in the spaces provided.

      a.   Frontal Eminences

      b.   Orbits

      c.   Nose

          (1)   Nares

          (2)   Nasal Septum

      d.   Philtrum

VII.   **Lateral Aspect of the Skull**

Describe these bones' articulations and landmarks of the lateral aspect of the skull.

    A.   **Bones**

1.   **Frontal Bone**

2.   **Parietal Bone**

3.   **Sphenoid Bone**

4.   **Temporal Bone**

   a.   **External Auditory Meatus**

   b.   **Mastoid Process**

   c.   **Styloid Process**

5.   Occipital Bone

B.   Articulations

Describe the locations of the following articulations of the skull bones. Include the names of the bones involved.

1.   Temporo-Zygomatic

2.   Pterion

VIII.   The Mandible

Describe these features of the mandible. Of what importance is the mandibular movement to normal speech?

A.   Importance in Speech

1.   Tongue Elevation

2.   Opening of the Oral Cavity

3.   **Point of Attachment for Muscles of Speech Articulation**

Identify the muscles of speech articulation that attach directly to the mandible.

B.   Importance in Deglutition

Describe the importance of the mandible to mastication.

1.   Opening of the Oral Cavity

2.   Mastication

Which muscles of mastication attach directly to the mandible?

C.   Structure of the Mandible

Describe the structure of the mandible in the spaces below.

1.   Corpus

a.   Mental Symphysis and Protuberance

b.   Inferior Alveolar Arch

Of what importance are the mandibular teeth to speech?

2.   Ramus

a.   Condylar Process

b.   Temporomandibular Joint

Describe the origins and insertions of the muscles that elevate the mandible. Which muscles depress the mandible? When are they used?

c.   Coronoid Process

What muscle attaches to the coronoid process?

d.   Angle of the Mandible

How does the angle of the mandible change as the individual develops?

IX.   The Speech Articulators

A.   Overview

1.   Form

Describe the structures and locations of the fixed and mobile speech articulators. State their roles in the production of specific obstruent consonants.

a.   Fixed Articulators

(1)   Upper Incisors

(2)   Superior Alveolar Ridge

(3)   Hard Palate (Maxillae)

b.   Mobile Articulators

(1)   Lips

(2)   Mandible

(3)   Soft Palate (Velum)

(4)   Tongue

(5)   Pharyngeal Walls

(6)   Larynx

2.   Function in Speech

Describe how the speech articulators perform the following functions in the production of phonemes.

a.   Modulation of Airflow for Consonant Articulation

b.   Alteration of Resonance for Vowel and Semivowel Articulation

3.   Function in Deglutition

Describe how the orofacial muscles perform the following functions in the intake of food and liquid.

a.   Retention of Material in Oral Cavity

b.   Sealing of Oral Cavity for Pressure Change

c.   Mastication

d.   Transfer of Bolus

e.   Protection of Airway

B. Oral Speech Articulators in Detail

Describe these details of the oral speech articulators in the spaces provided.

1. Extraoral (Facial) Articulators

a. Lips

(1) Vermilion Zone

(2) "Cupid's Bow"

(3) Effects of Lip Rounding

b. Muscles of Facial Expression

Describe the origins and insertions of these muscles. Describe the effects of their contraction.

(1) Sphincteric Muscles

(a)   **Orbicularis Oris**

(b)   **Orbicularis Oculi**

(2)   **Horizontal Muscles**

(a)   **Buccinator**

(b)   **Risorius**

(3)   **Angular Muscles**

(a)   Levator Labii Superiorus

(b)   Levator Labii Superiorus Alaeque Nasi

(c)   Zygomaticus Major

(d)   Zygomaticus Minor

(e)   Depressor Labii Inferiorus

(4)   Vertical Muscles

(a)   Mentalis

(b)   Depressor Anguli Oris

(c)   Levator Anguli Oris

(5)   Parallel Muscles

(a)   Incisivus Labii Superiorus

(b)   Incisivus Labii Inferiorus

Draw lines representing the courses of the fibers of the muscles of facial expression in the box below. Indicate the names of the muscles you are representing.

c. **Function of Extraoral Articulators**

(1) **Labial Consonants**

List the labial consonants using the International Phonetic Alphabet.

(2) **Rounded Vowels**

List the rounded vowels of American English. Is lip rounding associated with articulation of any consonants?

(3)   Gestural Communication

(4)   Retention of Fluids

d.   Motor Innervation

What is the major peripheral (cranial) nerve through which motor innervation of these muscles is provided?

e.   Sensory Innervation

Through which major peripheral (cranial) nerve are sensations of pain, temperature, and touch conveyed from the face to the central nervous system?

2.   Intraoral Articulators

Describe the form and functions of the following intraoral structures. What are their roles in the articulation of speech?

a.   Roof of the Oral Cavity

What are the possible effects of an unrepaired fistula (cleft) of the roof of the oral cavity?

(1)   Maxilla (Hard Palate)

(a)   Tissue Type

(b)   Superior Alveolar Ridge

(c)   Upper Dental Arch

(2)   Velum (Soft Palate)

(a)   Uvula

(b)   Velopharyngeal Sphincter

i) **Muscles of the Velopharyngeal Sphincter**

a) **Tensor Veli Palatini**

b) **Levator Veli Palatini**

c) **Palatopharyngeus**

d)   **Palatoglossus**

ii)   **Function of the Velopharyngeal
Sphincter**

iii)   **Motor Innervation**

Which peripheral nerves convey motor impulses from the central nervous system to the velopharyngeal sphincter muscles?

Draw a schematic representation of midsagittal view of the oral cavity in the box above. Include the lips, tongue, upper teeth, and the velum.

b.   **Floor of the Oral Cavity**

(1)   **The Tongue**

Describe the role of the tongue in the articulation of speech. List the consonants produced by articulation of the tongue with the other oral structures. Describe the role of the tongue in the articulation of vowels.

Draw a schematic representation of the open oral cavity as seen from the anterior aspect. Include the lips, tongue, upper teeth, and the velum.

(a)   Gross Structure of the Tongue

    i)   Parts of the Tongue

        a)   Apex

        b)   Dorsum

Front

Back

        c)   Blade

        d)   Root

ii)   Tissue Type of the Tongue

iii)   Landmarks of the Tongue

iv)   Attachments of the Tongue

v)   Intrinsic Muscles of the Tongue

a) Vertical

b) Transverse

c) Superior Longitudinal

d) Inferior Longitudinal

vi) Extrinsic Muscles of the Tongue

a) Genioglossus

b) Styloglossus

c) Hyoglossus

d)   Palatoglossus

vii)   **Motor Innervation of the Tongue**

viii)   **Sensory Innervation of the Tongue**

What is the role of the touch and stretch receptors of the tongue in the treatment of articulatory disorders? Do taste receptors have a role in the treatment of swallowing disorders?

a)   Touch

b)   Taste

c.   Posterior Oral Cavity

(1)   Faucial Pillars

(a)   Palatoglossus

(b)   Palatopharyngeus

(c)   Tonsillar Fossa

(2)   Tonsils (Waldeyer's Ring)

(a)   Functions

(b)   **Relevance to Speech Pathology**

(3)   **Posterior (Oro-) Pharyngeal Wall**

What functions do the posterior oral and pharyngeal structures have in modifying the quality of the speech signal?

(a)   **Superior and Middle Pharyngeal Constrictors**

(b)   **Passavant's Pad**

d.   Functions of Intraoral Articulators

In the box above, draw a midsagittal view of the oral cavity. Show the tongue, hard palate, and velum in the closed position.

X.   Deglutition

A.   Three Stages of Deglutition

Describe the progress of a bolus of food during each of these stages of deglutition

1.   Oral Stage (Voluntary)

a.   Preparation of the Bolus

b.   Elevation of Oral Floor

c.   Posterior Propulsion of Bolus

d.   Constriction of Posterior Oral Cavity

e.   Closing of Velopharyngeal Sphincter

2. Pharyngeal Stage (Involuntary)

    a.   Approximation of Aryepiglottic Folds

    b.   Arytenoid Cartilages Drawn Superiorly and Anteriorly

    c.   Elevation of Larynx and Articulation of Epiglottis

3. Esophageal Stage (Involuntary)

1. Which part of the skull includes the calvarium and the facial skeleton?

   _____.

2. A person viewing the skull from the lateral aspect would see which bones?

   _____.

3. The cheeks are formed by which bones? _____.

4. The mental protuberance is part of which bone? _____.

5. What are the three cavities of the vocal tract? _____, _____

   and _____.

6. Name the cavities of the cranium. _____.

7. The frontal bone forms which facial structure? _____.

8. Which muscles elevate the posterior part of the tongue? _____.

9. Which of the following are *mobile* articulators?

   a) Tongue;   b) Teeth;   c) Alveolar Ridge;   d) Velum;   e) Lips

10. A fistula between the oral and nasal cavities is commonly called a

    _____.

11. Which facial muscle(s) contract(s) when the speaker forms /u/?

    _____.

12. Which stage of deglutition is voluntary? _____.

13. Which muscles contract to elevate the mandible? _____.

14. Which articulators must function to produce /s/? _____.

ARTICULATORY SYSTEM

178

MUSCLES OF FACIAL EXPRESSION

FACIAL LANDMARKS

TEMPORALIS AND MASSETER MUSCLES

UNIT 6

THE NERVOUS SYSTEM

The nervous system is the medium by which the body realizes its wants and needs. Acting in concert with the endocrine system, the nervous system serves its function by virtue of the special conductivity and directionality of its constituent nervous tissue. The basic structure of the nervous system consists of the functional **neuron** and supportive **glial** tissues. The neuron consists of the **cell body** (soma), **axon**, **dendrite**, and the **synaptic junction**. It propagates ionic changes, called action potentials or neural impulses. These changes travel from the dendrites, past the cell body, to the axon. From there, they cross the cleft of the synapse to the next dendrite.

Anatomists divide the nervous system into central and peripheral systems, but these divisions are for convenience only. The nervous system functions as a whole.

The central nervous system consists of the **brain** and **spinal cord**. Both are contained in the axial skeleton, and are covered by three membranes, the meninges. The central nervous system mediates input from the peripheral nerves and effects its responses through them.

The brain is divided into two **hemispheres** connected by the **corpus callosum**. It contains more than twenty billion nerve cells and exercises executive control over higher mental sensory and motor functions. **Motor** and **sensory** functions of the right hemisphere are responsible for voluntary control and sensation on the left side of the body and vice versa. A **dominant hemisphere**, usually the left hemisphere, performs the crucial role in the reception and expression of language.

The gray **cerebral cortex** is a thin layer of cells covering the surface of the brain. It is a **convoluted** structure with **gyri** (ridges) and **sulci** (valleys) that serve as major anatomic landmarks for anatomists. Major sulci of the cortex include the **lateral**, **central**, and **calcarine** sulci. The major gyri of the cerebral cortex include the **precentral**, **postcentral**, **angular**, **supramarginal gyri**, and the **pars triangularis**. **Broca's** and **Wernicke's areas** are the major expressive and receptive speech and language centers, working in concert to perceive, formulate, express, and monitor spoken language.

There are four **lobes** of the cerebral cortex named after the bones of the skull under which they are located: **frontal**, **parietal**, **temporal**, and **occipital**. The neuronal tissue of all the cerebral lobes receive, relay, reverberate, store, and retrieve impulses from external and internal sources. None functions as an independent unit. The personality of an individual is the result of the combined functioning of all parts of the nervous system. The frontal lobe is the largest and forms the anterior portion of the hemisphere. The motor cortex and Broca's area are located in the frontal lobe. The **fissure of Rolando** or **central sulcus** divides the frontal and parietal lobes. The **primary motor cortex** lies immediately anterior to the central sulcus and the **primary sensory cortex** is posterior to this major landmark. The parietal lobe, forming the superior lateral portion of the hemisphere, is associated with the interpretation of sensory information. The **angular** and **supramarginal gyri** are also located in the parietal lobe. These gyri are associated with the interpretation of symbolic stimuli. The temporal lobe comprises the inferior lateral section of the hemisphere. It is associated with the interpretation of auditory input. The **auditory cortex** or **Heschl's gyrus** is located in the temporal lobe. The **fissure of Sylvius**, or **lateral sulcus**, separates the temporal and frontal lobes.

At the posterior region of the brain, the occipital lobe is delineated by the **lunate sulci**, visible on the medial surfaces of the hemispheres. The **primary visual cortex** is found in the occipital lobe. The **insular cortex** is sometimes identified as a cerebral lobe. It is located deep to the lateral fissure and is only visible by separating the bordering cortical tissue.

The interior of the brain contains the **white matter** and is made up of **afferent** and **efferent projection fibers**. White fibers are so called because they are sheathed in a white fatty **myelin sheath**. They converge at the **internal capsules** and **thalami** of each hemisphere, and descend through the **midbrain**, **pons**, and **medulla** levels of the **brainstem**. The white matter also contains commissural and association fibers that connect centers within and between the cerebral hemispheres.

Four **ventricles**, cavities filled with **cerebrospinal fluid**, are deep within the white matter. Cerebrospinal fluid is created in these ventricles and flows out and around the central nervous system. The fluid protects the central nervous system and helps regulate intracranial pressure.

The circulation of blood is critical to brain function. Neuronal tissues die very shortly after interruption in their ability to perform metabolism. Central nervous system neurons have very limited regenerative ability and are generally replaced with structural **glial** tissue after they die. The **internal carotid** and **vertebral arteries** supply blood to the brain. They conjoin at the **circle of Willis** where **anterior**, **posterior**, and **middle** cerebral arteries provide the primary blood supply to the hemispheres. Venous drainage is provided by the **dural sinuses** and the **jugular veins**.

The **spinal cord** is the caudal extension of the brainstem. It is the major conduit for impulses passing to or from the central nervous system and the peripheral nervous system. The spinal cord, as a central nervous system structure, processes some reflexive neural information. Spinal cord functions are said to be **segmental**.

The peripheral nervous system consists of the **12 cranial nerves**, **31 spinal nerves**, and the **autonomic nervous system**. The cranial nerves have synaptic connections with the brainstem. They are final common pathways for most of the sensory and motor functions of the peripheral speech and hearing mechanisms. Spinal nerves synapse at nuclei at or very close to the spinal cord. The autonomic nervous system has both **sympathetic** and **parasympathetic** divisions that maintain and regulate unconscious bodily functions or adapt them in emergencies.

The objectives for this unit are to provide the student a foundation for further study of this vastly complex subject. Students should mark progress by checking the boxes beside each objective as they accomplish them.

1. Describe the general organization of the human nervous system.

2. Differentiate between afferent and efferent functions.

3. Describe the major components of the central nervous system.

4. Name the major parts of the human brain.

5. Name and describe the general functions of the lobes of the cerebral cortex.

6. Identify, using diagrams or models, the major landmarks of the cerebral cortex and describe their general functions.

7. Identify, using diagrams, the major subcortical structures of the brain and describe their major functions.

8. Identify and describe the general function of the cerebellum.

9. Name and describe the three meninges and their relative locations.

10. Describe the flow of cerebrospinal fluid.

11. Describe the major components of the peripheral nervous system.

12. Name and describe the communication functions of the cranial nerves.

13. Name and describe some commonly encountered syndromes associated with disorders of the human nervous system.

I.   General Organization of the Human Nervous System

Describe the overall organization of the human nervous system. How do the two major divisions serve each other? Is it realistic to consider the system as composed of two separate entities?

A.   Basic Structures

1.   The Neuron

a.   Cell Body

b.   Axon

c.   Dendrite

d.   Synapses

2.   **Glial Tissue**

B.   **Central Nervous System**

Describe the locations and general functions of the major parts of the central nervous system.

1.   **Brain**

a.   Cerebral Hemispheres

(1)   Cerebral Cortex

(a)   Location

(b)   General Function

(2)   Subcortical Structures

(a)   Location

(b)   General Function

b. Brainstem

(1) Location

(2) General Function

c. Cerebellum

(1) Location

(2) General Function

2. Spinal Cord

a.   Location

b.   General Function

C.   Peripheral Nervous System

1.   Spinal and Cranial Nerves

Give the general locations of the nuclei of the cranial and the spinal nerves. Describe the general differences in functions between the cranial nerves and the spinal nerves.

a.   12 Cranial Nerves

b. 31 Spinal Nerves

2. Autonomic Nervous System (Ganglia and Nerve Processes)

Describe the general differences between the sympathetic and parasympathetic divisions of the autonomic nervous system

a. Sympathetic Division

b. Parasympathetic Division

II. The Brain in Detail

Describe the form and functions of these structures of the brain.

A. Cerebral Hemispheres

1.   Cerebral Cortex

    a.   Structure of the Cerebral Cortex

        (1)   Major Sulci of the Cerebral Cortex

            (a)   Lateral Sulcus (Fissure of Sylvius)

                i)   Location of the Lateral Sulcus

                ii)   Insula

iii)   Opercula

iv)   Parallel Sulcus

(b)   Central Sulcus (Fissure of Rolando)

i)   Location of the Central Sulcus

ii)   Precentral and Postcentral Functions

(c)   Calcarine Fissure

(2)   Major Gyri of the Cerebral Cortex

Describe the locations of these gyri of the cerebral cortex.

(a)   **Precentral gyrus**

(b)   **Postcentral Gyrus**

(c)   **Angular Gyrus**

(d)   **Supramarginal Gyrus**

(e)   **Pars Triangularis**

b.   General Functions of Areas of the Cerebral Cortex

Describe the locations of these specific areas of the cerebral cortex. Draw their locations in the space provided.

(1)   Sensory Cortex

(2)   Motor Cortex

(3)   Auditory Cortex

(4)   Visual Cortex

2.   Hemispheric Functions

a.   Interhemispheric Differences

(1)   Cerebral Dominance

What is meant by "cerebral dominance?"

(a)   Incidence of Left or Right Hemisphere Dominance

(b)   Relationship to Handedness

(2)   Dominant Hemisphere Functions

(3)   Nondominant Hemisphere Functions

b.   Interhemispheric Communication

Name and locate the major interhemispheric connections.

c.   Intrahemispheric Communication

Name and locate the major intrahemispheric communication pathways.

3.   Lobes of the Cerebral Cortex

Describe the forms and functions of the following structures of the cerebral cortex.

a.   Frontal Lobe

(1)   Location

(2)   Functions

Describe and name the possible effects of a lesion in the following locations.

(a)   Motor Cortex (Precentral Gyrus)

i)   Homunculus (Projections)

ii)   Decussation of Motor Tracts

(b)   Association Areas

i)   Premotor Cortex

ii)   Broca's Area (Pars Triangularis)

(c)   Other Functions

b.   Parietal Lobe

(1)   Location

(a)   Postcentral Gyrus

(b)   Somesthetic Cortex (Sensory Cortex)

(2)   Functions
Describe the possible effects of a lesion in the following locations.

(a)   Sensory Decussation

(b)   Sensory Homunculus

(c)   Stereognosis

Define stereognosis. What role does stereognosis play in the production (or perception) of speech?

(3)   Angular Gyrus

What effect might a lesion in this area have on communication?

(4)   Supramarginal Gyrus

What effect might a lesion in this area have on communication?

c.   Temporal Lobe

(1)   Location

(a)   Temporal Gyri

(b)   Auditory Cortex (Heschl's Gyri)

(2)   Functions

Describe and name the possible effects of a temporal lobe lesion on the following functions.

(a)   Sensation

(b)   Perception

(c)   Association

(3)   Wernicke's Area

Describe where this area is located and explain the potential effects of a lesion in this area on communication.

d.   Occipital Lobe

(1)   Location

(a)   Parieto-Occipital Fissure

(b)   Calcarine Fissure

(c)   Visual Cortex

(2)   Functions

Describe and name the possible effects of a lesion on the following occipital lobe functions.

(a)   Sensation

i)   Retinal Projections

ii)   Optic Decussation

What is a "decussation?" Be alert for other examples of decussation in the central nervous system.

iii)   Anopsia

(b)   Perception

(c)   Association

4.   **Subcortical Structures**

Describe the locations and functions of these subcortical structures in the spaces provided. Indicate the structures for which researchers have yet to reveal clear roles. Describe the possible effects of lesions in the following areas.

a.   **Thalamus**

(1)   Location

(2)   Structure

(3)   Function

b.   Hypothalamus

c.   Pineal Body

d.   Basal Nuclei (Striate Bodies)

(1)   Names

(2)   General Location

(3)   Structure

(4)   Functions

What effect might a lesion in this area have on communication?

5.   **Brainstem**

Draw a schematic representation of the brainstem and label the three major divisions.

a.   **Location**

(1)   **Midbrain**

(2)   **Pons**

(3)   **Medulla**

b.   **Relationship to Spinal Cord**

c.   **Functions**

Briefly describe these central nervous system functions aggregated in the brainstem.

(1)   Ascending/Descending Tracts (CNS)

(a)   Decussations

i)   **Motor**

ii)   **Sensory**

a)   **Pyramidal**

b)   **Extrapyramidal**

ii)   Sensory

a)   Spinothalamic Tracts

b)   Trigeminothalamic Tracts

(b)   Reticular System

(c)   Vestibular System

6.   Cerebellum

a.   Location

b.   Function

7.   Meninges

a.   Dura

b.   Arachnoid

c.   Pia

8.   Cerebrospinal Fluid (CSF)

a.   Composition

Describe the composition of cerebrospinal fluid.

b.   Function

What are the functions of cerebrospinal fluid?

c.   Ventricles

Where are the four ventricles?

d.   Foramina

How does CSF flow from one ventricle to another?

e.   Subarachnoid Space

f.   Flow of Cerebrospinal Fluid

Describe the production, flow, and absorption of CSF in the space below.

III.   Spinal Cord in Detail

A.   Structure

Describe the extent and sections of the spinal cord.

B.   **Function**

What is the function of the spinal cord?

IV.   **Peripheral Nervous System**

A.   **Spinal and Cranial Nerves**

Describe the differences in locations and functions between the cranial nerves and the spinal nerves.

1.   **12 Cranial Nerves**

Beside each cranial nerve name, write its communicative function(s). Use the letters "S," "M," or "B" to indicate if the nerve has "sensory," "motor ," or "both" functions.

a.   I Olfactory

b.   II Optic

c.   III Oculomotor

d.   IV Trochlear

e.   V Trigeminal

f.   VI Abducens

g.   VII Facial

h.   **VIII Vestibulocochlear**

i.   **IX Glossopharyngeal**

j.   **X Vagus**

k.   **XI Accessory**

l.   **XII Hypoglossal**

2.   **31 Spinal Nerves**

Where are the spinal nerves located? What communicative functions do the spinal nerves have?

B.   Autonomic Nervous System (Ganglia and Nerve Processes)

Describe the general differences between the sympathetic and parasympathetic divisions of the autonomic nervous system

1.   Sympathetic

   a.   Thoracolumbar Outflow

   b.   Emergency Actions

2.   Parasympathetic

   a.   Craniosacral Outflow

   b.   Normal Bodily Functions

1. What are the two main divisions of the human nervous system?

    _____ and _____.

2. The central nervous system is composed of _____ and _____.

3. Sensory input is carried over _____ tracts.

4. Motor impulses are carried over _____ tracts.

5. The primary motor cortex is located in the _____ lobe.

6. There are _____ pairs of cranial nerves.

7. The spinal nerves are parts of the nervous _____ system.

8. The peripheral nervous system is subdivided into which parts?

    _____.

9. The emergency acceleration in heart rate and increased perspiration, which accompany the presence of anxiety-evoking stimuli is accomplished through action of: _____.

10. The recognition that the (above) anxiety-evoking stimuli are present is mediated by _____.

11. Nerves connect to one another at _____.

12. The raised portions of the convoluted surface of the cerebral hemispheres are called _____.

13. The temporal lobe is separated from the parietal and frontal lobes by

    _____.

14. The precentral and postcentral gyri are separated by

    _____.

15. The gyrus immediately posterior to the central sulcus is attributed with the

    function of _____.

16. Broca's area is located in the _____.

17. What condition will result when the visual cortex of one cerebral hemisphere is

    destroyed? _____.

18. A unilateral lesion of the motor cortex of the right hemisphere will result in

    _____.

19. The midbrain, pons, and medulla are parts of the _____.

20. The intrinsic muscles of the tongue receive their motor innervation via which

    cranial nerve? _____.

NERVOUS SYSTEM

223

UNIT 7

THE AUDITORY SYSTEM

The process of hearing depends on the transmission and transformation of energy. **Acoustic** energy must pass through three media and be converted into the **electro-chemical** energy of the nervous system before the listener becomes aware of its presence. The clarity with which the sound is heard depends on the successful transmission of vibration energy from air to body tissues, and then to fluid.

Sound begins as the disruption of random molecular movements in a **medium**, usually air, by the directed displacements of a vibrating body. The vibrating body is referred to as the **source**.

Molecules in all matter are simultaneously attracted to and repelled from one another by the atomic forces of their components. The source applies additional force to adjacent molecules, and a chain reaction begins. Thus, the sound is **propagated**. Each displaced molecule in the medium absorbs some of the energy exerted upon it, but passes the residual energy on to nearby molecules. The process by which the molecules approach each other and bounce back is known as **compression** and **rarefaction**. Compression occurs when the distance between molecules is decreased and rarefaction occurs when the distance between the molecules is greater than during the normal state.

The listener becomes aware of the presence of sound when air molecules near the ear are set into motion with characteristics resembling those of the source. The sound must be of sufficient strength, or **intensity**, and within the anatomically determined range of **frequencies** to be transmitted by the ear and detected by the brain.

The **pinna** channels acoustic energy into the middle ear. The **external auditory meatus**, in its normal anatomic form, enhances sounds within the acoustic range of speech, and protects the sensitive deep structures of the auditory system. The external meatus leads to the **tympanic membrane**. The tympanic membrane divides the outer and **middle ear** and vibrates at a frequency and amplitude corresponding to the molecular displacements in the external meatus.

Sound energy passes on to the **middle ear**, or **tympanum**. The middle ear is an aspirin-sized cavity in the temporal bones of the skull. Because the cavity is closed at each end, a **eustachian tube** passes from within to the nasopharynx. This tube serves to equalize air pressure when required. Secured to the tympanic membrane are the three tiny bones of the middle ear known as the **ossicles: malleus, incus**, and **stapes**. These bones vibrate in unison with the tympanic membrane and amplify the energy transmitted to the inner ear.

The **inner ear** contains the sensory end organ of hearing, the **cochlea**. The cochlea is part of a complex sensory structure called the **labyrinth**. The labyrinth is so named because it consists of soft tissue organs embedded in a series of tunnels hollowed out of the temporal bone of the skull. The cochlear tunnel is snail-shaped. Here, the medium of sound transmission becomes a fluid called **endolymph**. The fluid within the cochlea is set into vibration, which in turn, sets the **organ of Corti** on the **basilar membrane** into vibration. This vibration occurs at a frequency and amplitude corresponding to the ossicular chain vibration. Attached to the organ of Corti are epithelial **hair cells**, connected to the nerve endings of the **spiral ganglion**. Each hair cell movement sets off a subsequent neurologic impulse along the **vestibulocochlear** or **eighth cranial nerve**. At this stage of the hearing process, the hydraulic energy occurring in the cochlea transforms into nerve or electrochemical energy.

The vestibulocochlear nerve enters the brainstem at a structure called the **medulla**. From the medulla, some nerve fibers enter a structure known as the **thalamus**. It is the thalamus, in combination with other brain structures that regulates which auditory signals are attended to and which are ignored. From the thalamus, the electrochemical energy is transmitted upward to the cortex where interpretation of the sound occurs.

Another sensory structure of the labyrinth is the **vestibular system**. This system senses the pull of gravity on its receptors. Its nerve endings interact with the body's axial and appendicular skeletal muscles and with the extraocular eye muscles. The vestibular system helps the body maintain its posture through the sense of balance. It consists of the **utricle**, the **saccule**, and three **semicircular canals**.

Objectives for this unit are intended to orient the student to the fundamental form and function of the auditory system. With such preparation, the student should be ready to pursue further study in either audiology, speech-language pathology, or related fields. Students should check the boxes beside each objective to mark their progress toward that overall goal.

✐ ☐ 1. Identify and describe the functions of the two main divisions of the human auditory system.

✐ ☐ 2. Describe the structures of the human auditory system as being located in the peripheral or central divisions of the auditory system.

✐ ☐ 3. Identify the anatomic limits and describe the functions of the peripheral hearing mechanism.

✐ ☐ 4. Name the three main parts of the peripheral hearing mechanism.

✐ ☐ 5. Describe the structures of the peripheral hearing mechanism as being located in the external, middle, or inner ear(s).

✐ ☐ 6. Locate the major landmarks of the pinna.

✐ ☐ 7. Name and describe the morphologies and locations of the ossicles.

✐ ☐ 8. Describe the major functions of the parts of the peripheral hearing mechanism, including:

a. the pinna	f. the ossicles
b. the external auditory meatus	g. the cochlea
c. the tympanic membrane	h. the vestibule
d. the tympanum	i. the semicircular canals
e. the eustachian tubes	j. the vestibulocochlear nerve

✐ ☐ 9. Identify and describe the functions of the following structures of the cochlea:

a. scala media	g. organ of Corti
b. scala tympani	h. hair cells
c. scala vestibuli	i. Reissner's membrane
d. basilar membrane	j. endolymph
e. tectorial membrane	k. perilymph
f. auditory nerve	l. helicotrema

✎ ☐ 10. Identify the anatomic limits and describe the functions of the central auditory system.

✎ ☐ 11. Describe, in sequence, the transmission of auditory evoked potentials with respect to the following central auditory system structures:

   a. cochlear nuclei
   b. superior olivary complex
   c. medial geniculate body of the thalamus
   d. cerebral cortex

I. Two Main Divisions of the Human Auditory System

Describe the location and functions of the two main divisions of the human auditory system.

A. Peripheral Auditory System

1. Location and Extent

2. Functions

B. Central Auditory System

1. Location and Extent

2. Functions

II. The Peripheral Hearing Mechanism in Detail

Describe the forms (extent) and functions of the following structures of the peripheral hearing mechanism in the spaces provided.

A. External (Outer) Ear

1. Pinna (Auricle)

a. Form

Locate the following parts of the pinna and label them on the illustration (on page 259).

231

(1)   Helix

(2)   Antihelix

(3)   Tragus

(4)   Antitragus

(5)   Lobe

(6)   Concha

(7)   Triangular Fossa

b.   Functions of the Pinna

What are the hearing functions of the pinna? Does the pinna have functions other than those for hearing?

2.   External Auditory Meatus (EAM)

a.   Form

(1)   Ear Canal

(a)   Shape

(b)   **Underlying Tissue Composition**

(c)   **Cerumen**

What are the origin and purposes of cerumen?

(2)   **Tympanic Membrane**

Is the tympanic membrane part of the outer or middle ear? In the spaces below describe the parts of the tympanic membrane and their functions.

(a)   **Laminae**

(b)   **Pars Tensa**

(c)   **Pars Flaccida**

(d)   **Otoscopic Landmarks**

Draw a schematic representation of the tympanic membrane as seen from the external auditory meatus in the box below. Label the following landmarks.

   i)   **Pars Tensa**

   ii)   **Pars Flaccida**

   iii)   **Malleolar Stria**

b.   Functions

Describe the functions of the external ear in the spaces provided.

(1)   Acoustic Function

(2)   Protective Function

c.   Mastoid Process (of Temporal Bone)

How do audiologists use the mastoid process to specify the natures of hearing disorders?

B.   Middle Ear (Tympanum)

Describe these aspects of the middle ear in the spaces provided.

1.   General Form and Extent

2. Function

3. Structures of the Middle Ear

    a. Tympanic Membrane

        (1) Structure

        Describe the laminae of the tympanic membrane.

        (2) Function

    b. Ossicles

        (1) Form

        In the box on the right, draw a stylized diagram of the relationship of the ossicular chain to the tympanic membrane and to the oval window. Label each ossicle.

(a)   Malleus

(b)   Incus

(c)   Stapes

(2)   Impedance Matching Function

*Describe two ways the ossicular chain matches
acoustic impedance between the atmosphere and
the cochlear fluids.*

c.   Eustachian (Pharyngotympanic) Tubes

(1)   Structure and Location

(2)   Function

d.   Muscles of the Middle Ear

(1)   Stapedius

(2)   Tensor Tympani

(3)   Acoustic Reflex

Does the acoustic reflex serve a protective function?

4.   **Middle Ear Function Testing**

Describe how audiologists test the function of the middle ear. Why is the otoscope an important tool in the examination of the peripheral hearing mechanism?

C.   **Inner Ear (Labyrinth)**

1.   **Location**

In what portion of the temporal bone is the inner ear located?

2.   **Bony Labyrinth**

3.   **Membranous Labyrinth**

4.   **Inner Ear Structures**

    a.   **Hearing Mechanism**

        (1)   **Cochlea**

            (a)   **Shape**

            Describe the shape of the cochlea. How many turns does it make from basal to apical ends?

                i)   **Basal End**

                ii)   **Apical End**

            (b)   **Membranous Portion of the Cochlea**

i)   **Scala Media**

Where are these fluids found relative to the scala media?

a)   **Endolymph**

b)   **Perilymph**

ii)   **Basilar Membrane**

Describe these structures of the basilar membrane.

a)   **Organ of Corti**

b)   **Hair Cells**

c)   **Tectorial Membrane**

d)   **Spiral Ganglion**

iii)   **Reissner's (Vestibular) Membrane**

(c)   **Bony Portion of the Cochlea**

Describe the locations of these structures of the bony portion of the cochlea. What hearing function do these structures play?

i)   **Scala Tympani**

ii)   Scala Vestibuli

iii)   Helicotrema

iv)   Modiolus

(2)   **Cochlear Nerve**

What is the other division of the eighth cranial nerve?

(a)   **VIIIth Cranial Nerve: Auditory Division**

(b)   **Cochlear Nuclei**

(c)   **Cochlear Nuclear Synapses**

b.   Vestibular Mechanism (System)

Describe these structures of the vestibular mechanism. What is the general function of this mechanism?

(1)   Utricle

(2)   Saccule

(3)   Central Structure of Labyrinth

(4)   Semicircular Canals

(a)   Vertical Canals

i)   Anterior

ii)   Posterior

(b)   Horizontal Canal

c.   Inner Ear Functions

(1)   Functions for Hearing Mechanism

(a)   Basilar Membrane

i)   Frequency Analysis

ii)   Transduction

How does the basilar membrane act as an energy transducer?

(b)   Auditory Nerve

i)   Threshold

Define threshold as it applies to auditory testing.

ii)   **Firing Rate of the Nerve**

How does firing rate of the acoustic nerve relate to the listener's perception of loudness?

iii)   **Frequency Perception**

What is the current theory regarding the role of the auditory nerve in frequency perception?

iv)   **Temporal Perception**

What is meant by "temporal perception?"

(2)   **Functions of Vestibular Mechanism**

Describe the significance of these aspects of vestibular function.

(a)   **Perception of Position in Space**

(b)   Relationship to Extraocular Muscles

(c)   Relationship to Muscles of Posture and Locomotion

III.   The Central Auditory System

In the spaces provided, describe these anatomic aspects of the central auditory system.

A.   Location and Limits

B.   Structures of the Central Auditory System

1.   Brainstem Structures

a.   Pons

b. Midbrain

2. Thalamus

What other special senses have relay centers in the thalamus?

3. Cerebral Cortex

a. Heschl's Gyrus

b. Association Areas

C.   **Functions of the Central Auditory System: The Central Auditory Pathways**

Describe the course of auditory stimuli from the cochlea to the cerebral cortex via the structures listed below. How are these action potentials tracked? How do audiologists employ such tracking for diagnostic purposes? Describe any role physiologists think it may have in refining the listener's perception of auditory stimuli.

1.   Brainstem

    a.   Pons

        (1)   Cochlear Nuclei

    (a)   **Dorsal Cochlear Nucleus**

    (b)   **Ventral Cochlear Nucleus**

        i)   **Anteroventral Cochlear Nucleus**

        ii)   **Posteroventral Cochlear Nucleus**

    (c)   **Tonotopic Representation**

What is tonotopic representation?

(2)   **Superior Olivary Complex**

    (a)   **Decussation**

    (b)   Localization of Sound Source

    (c)   Olivocochlear Tracts

b.   **Midbrain**

    (1)   **Lateral Lemniscus**

    (a)   Inferior Colliculus

    (b)   Nucleus of the Lateral Lemniscus

(c)   Olivocochlear Bundle Fibers

How do audiologists use action potentials from the olivocochlear fibers to evaluate cochlear functions?

(2)   Association with Other Functions

2.   Thalamus

a.   Location

b.   General Function

(1)   Sensory

(2)   Emotional

c.   Medial Geniculate Body

3.   Cerebral Cortex

Does the cerebral cortex appear to deal differently with meaningful auditory stimuli than it does with nonmeaningful ones?

a.   Temporal Lobe

(1)   Heschl's Gyrus

(2)   Association Areas

(3)   Interaction with Other Cortical Functions

Describe the way auditory signals are associated with signals from other input modalities at the level of the cerebral cortex.

b.   Interhemispheric Differences

(1)   Sensation

(2)   Perception

Describe what is meant by "perception." Are there different levels of perception?

(a)   Interhemispheric Differences in Auditory Perception

i)   Perception of Speech

ii)   Perception of Other Stimuli

(3)   Auditory Discrimination

(a)   Of General Acoustic Stimuli

(b)   **Of Speech Stimuli**

(4)   **Auditory Memory**

1. The external auditory meatus is part of the _____.

2. What is the major contribution of the pinna to hearing?

    _____.

3. The skeleton of the distal portion of the external auditory meatus is composed

    of _____.

4. The main function of the middle ear is _____.

5. The ossicular chain is composed of which three bones?

    _____.

6. Pressure equalization for the middle ear is provided by

    _____.

7. The semicircular canals are parts of the _____.

8. The end organ for hearing is the _____.

9. With what fluid are scala vestibuli and scala tympani filled? _____.

10. The cranial nerve that carries sound-activated nerve impulses to the brainstem

    is _____.

11. The cranial nerves connect to the central nervous system at what structure?

    _____.

12. Nerve fibers of the auditory pathways cross from one side of the brainstem to

    the contralateral side at the level of the _____.

13. In most people, meaningful language input is mediated primarily in the

    _____.

14. The auditory cortex is located in the _____.

15. The first synapses of the central auditory pathway are the

    _____.

16. A tumor that affects transmission of VIIIth nerve impulses is called

    _____.

17. Indicate in which division (central or peripheral) of the auditory system the

    following structures are located.

    a. stapedius muscle: _____.

    b. cochlea: _____.

    c. pinna: _____.

    d. dorsal cochlear nucleus: _____.

    e. inferior olive: _____.

    f. stapes: _____.

    g. ceruminous glands: _____.

    h. VIIIth nerve: _____.

    i. Heschl's gyrus: _____.

    j. organ of Corti: _____.

18. The semicircular canals are parts of what system/mechanism? _____.

19. Which ossicle is located closest to the tympanic membrane? _____.

20. What are the three main parts of the peripheral hearing mechanism?

    _____.

PINNA

CORONAL VIEW OF PERIPHERAL HEARING MECHANISM

REFERENCES AND RECOMMENDED READINGS

Anderson, K. (Ed.). (1994). *Mosby's medical, nursing, and allied health dictionary*. St.Louis: Mosby-Year Book.

Brookes, M., & Zeitman, A. (1998). *Clinical embryology: A color atlas of the human body*. Philadelphia: Lea & Febiger.

Clemente, C. (1975). *Anatomy: A regional atlas of the human body*. Philadelphia: Lea & Febiger.

Daniloff, R., Schuckers, G., & Feth, L. (1980). *The physiology of speech and hearing*. Englewood Cliffs, NJ: Prentice-Hall.

Goode, R., Killion, M., Nakamura, K., & Nishihara, S. (1994). New knowledge about the function of the human middle ear: Development of an improved analog model. *American Journal of Otology, 15,* 145–154.

Hafen, B., & Karren, K. (1989). *Prehospital emergency care and crisis intervention*. Englewood, CO: Morton Publishing.

Hamilton, W. (1977). *Textbook of human anatomy*. St. Louis, MO: C.V. Mosby.

Katz, J. (1994). *Handbook of clinical audiology*. Baltimore: Williams and Wilkins.

Larsen, W. J. (2001). *Clinical embryology* (3rd ed.). New York: Churchill Livingstone.

Martin, F. (1994). *Introduction to audiology* (5th ed.) Englewood Cliffs, NJ: Prentice-Hall.

Minifie, F., Hixon, T., & Williams, F. (1973). *Normal aspects of speech, hearing, and language*. Englewood Cliffs, NJ: Prentice-Hall.

Romanes, G. (Ed.). (1972). *Cunningham's textbook of anatomy* (11th ed.). London: Oxford University Press.

Thomas, C. (Ed.). (1973). *Taber's cyclopedic medical dictionary*. Philadelphia: F.A. Davis Company.

Van Riper, C., & Erickson, R. (1996). *Speech correction: An introduction to speech pathology and audiology* (9th ed.). Needham Heights, MA: Allyn & Bacon.

Von Bekesy, G. (1989). *Experiments in hearing*. New York: Acoustical Society of America.

Zemlin, W. (1998). *Speech and hearing science: Anatomy and physiology* (4th ed.). Englewood Cliffs, NJ: Prentice-Hall.

Zwislocki, J. J. (1975). The role of the external and middle ears in sound transmission. In H. Winitz (Ed.), *Human communication and its disorders: The nervous system* (Vol. 3, pp. 45–55). Greenwich, CT: Ablex Publishing.

ANSWERS TO SELF-TESTS

1. Erect, facing the observer; front; directed toward the observer; at the sides.

2. Physiology

3. Coronal

4. Transverse

5. Superior

6. Inferior or distal

7. Distal

8. Lateral

9. Inferior or distal

10. Anatomy

11. Geriatric

12. Developmental

13. Pathologic

14. Experimental

1.   Protoplasm.

2.   Growth; reproduction; metabolism; adaptation

3.   Histology.

4.   Nucleus.

5.   a) Nervous; b) Epithelial; c) Muscle; d) Connective; e) Nervous

6.   a) Ectoderm; b) Mesoderm; c) Ectoderm; d) Mesoderm;
     e) Endoderm (Entoderm).

7.   Mandible and hyoid bones; thyroid and cricoid cartilages

8.   Intake of food, water, and air.

9.   Germ layers

10. Diarthrodial or synovial

11. Striated or skeletal

12. A motor neuron and the muscle fibers it supplies.

13. Insertion

14. A collection of tissues that work together to perform a specific function.

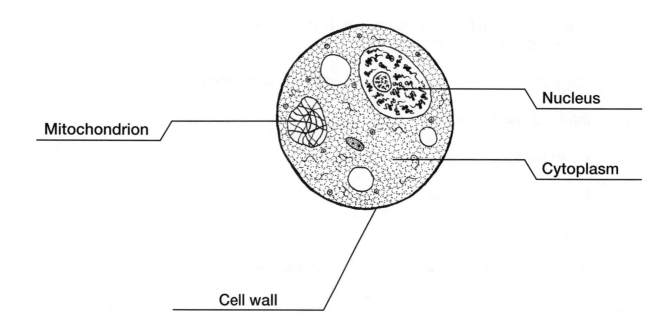

Mitochondrion

Nucleus

Cytoplasm

Cell wall

SOMATIC CELL

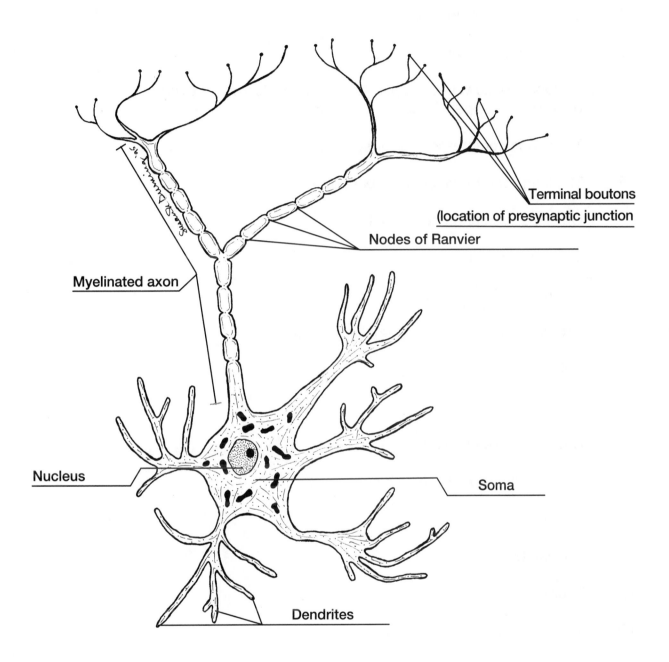

Terminal boutons
(location of presynaptic junction

Nodes of Ranvier

Myelinated axon

Nucleus

Soma

Dendrites

NEURON

1.   Chemical and Biological

2.   Volume; Boyle's Law.

3.   a. Upper; b. Lower; c. Upper; d. Upper; e. Upper; f. Lower;
     g. Lower; h. Upper; i. Lower; j. Upper

4.   To provide compressed air for speech

5.   The lungs and the respiratory passages

6.   One inhalation and one exhalation

7.   12 to 20 cycles/min.

8.   The muscles of respiration

9.   The diaphragm and the external intercostals

10. Relax

11. Cervical

12. Bucket-handle movement

13. Forced exhalation, such as blowing

14. Sternum

15. Spirometer

16. Thoracic

17. Tidal volume

18. Vital capacity

19. 0.16

20. Supplemental air; can be forcefully exhaled from resting expiratory level.

21. Diaphragmatic/abdominal; thoracic.

22. Rapid, shallow cycles (tachypnea) gradually becoming longer and deeper (hyperpnea), followed by transient cessation of breathing (apnea). After this, the pattern repeats.

23. Chronic obstructive pulmonary disease (COPD) is an irreversible condition in which the patient is unable to make optimal use of the oxygen in the air for respiration. Depending on the severity of the condition, the patient may be forced to speak in short utterances. Expiratory volume velocity may be insufficient to produce a normal voice. Because the condition is irreversible, rehabilitation goals should be aimed at accommodation instead of recovery.

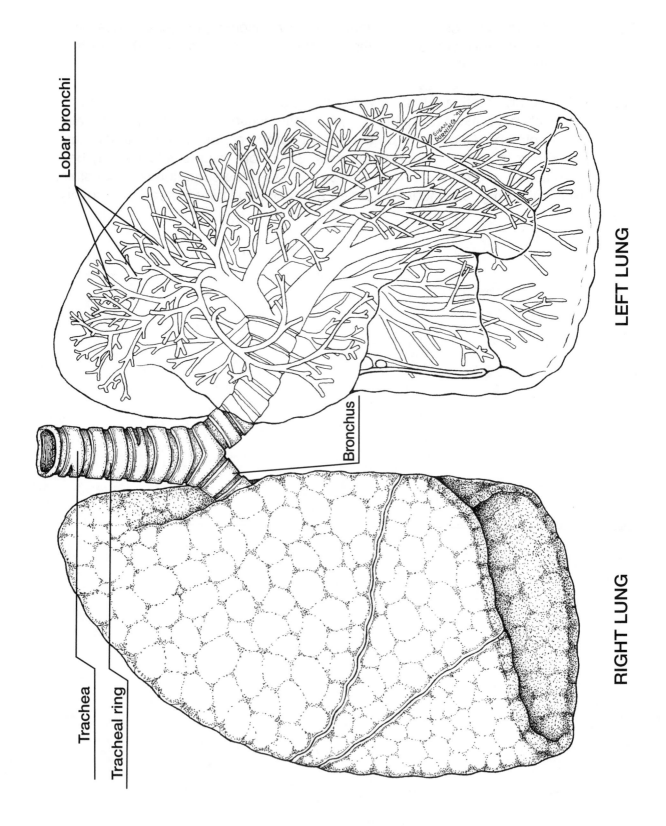

Lobar bronchi

LEFT LUNG

Bronchus

Trachea

Tracheal ring

RIGHT LUNG

6th cervical vertebra

1st rib

2nd rib

Sternum

External Intercostal muscles

Xiphoid process

Diaphragm

3rd lumbar vertebra

THORACIC SKELETON

271

1.   To protect the airway.

2.   Anterior

3.   To produce a phonatory source for speech.

4.   The complex tone produced when loosely approximated vocal folds emit pulses of pulmonary air.

5.   The number of times the glottis opens and closes in a given time.

6.   The amount of subglottic pressure

7.   The space between the vocal folds

8.   Skull

9.   The thyroid cartilage

10.   The cricoid cartilage

11.   Laminae (singular: lamina)

12.   "Adam's apple"

13.   Cricoid cartilage

14.   The vocal processes of the arytenoid cartilages

15.   Abduction

16.   (d) Cricothyroid, thyroarytenoid, and vocalis muscles

17.   (a) Posterior cricoarytenoid muscles

18.   The muscular processes of the arytenoid cartilages

19.   Abducted

20.   Synovial

21.   Vocal ligament

22. The intrinsic muscles are attached to laryngeal structures at both ends, while the extrinsic muscles are attached to laryngeal structures at one end and attached to other structures (i.e., the sternum) at the other end.

23. The posterior cricoarytenoids

24. To adjust the support, posture, and position of the larynx

25. Subglottic pressure

26. Approximately 210 Hz. (Some authorities give 260 Hz.)

27. During phonation the glottis closes through combined myoelastic and aerodynamic forces. Myoelasticity is the tendency of the muscles to resist deformation. Aerodynamic forces result from the Bernoulli effect, or the tendency of the internal pressure of a liquid (such as air) to decrease as its velocity increases.

28. The thyroarytenoid and vocalis muscles

29. Superiorly

30. Radiologists and speech-language pathologists perform videoflouroscopy or fiberoptic evaluations of the swallowing mechanism. Part of this evaluation requires watching for an abnormal collection of food or liquid material in the valleculae. Spillage of a portion of the bolus into the valleculae before a pharyngeal swallow is triggered may lead to aspiration of food or liquid material into the airway before the swallow. In addition the inability to clear food residue from the valleculae after the swallow may lead to aspiration of this food or liquid material after the swallow. Following the videoflouroscopic or fiberoptic evaluation, the functioning (or malfunctioning) at the level of the valleculae may lead to differing recommendations from the speech-language pathologist regarding a patient's ability to tolerate various food or liquid consistencies.

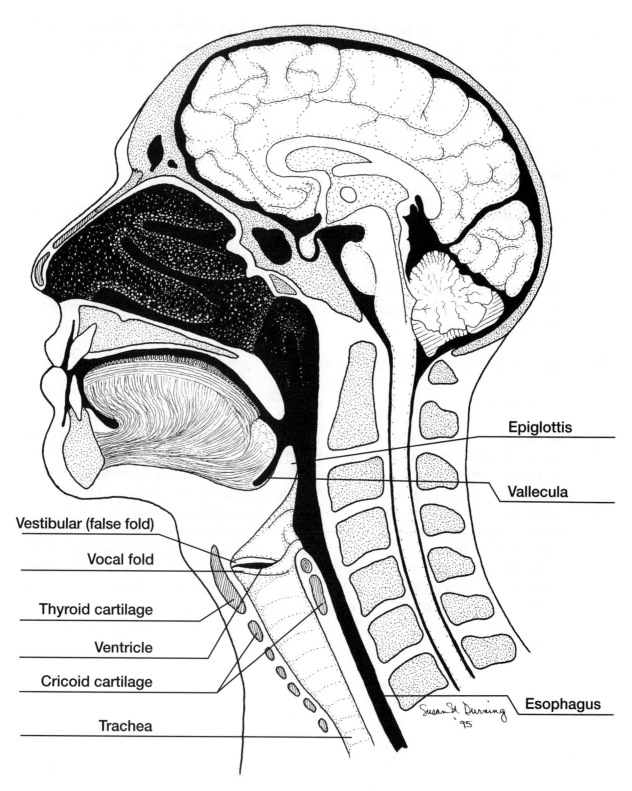

Epiglottis

Vallecula

Vestibular (false fold)

Vocal fold

Thyroid cartilage

Ventricle

Cricoid cartilage

Esophagus

Trachea

PHONATORY SYSTEM

274

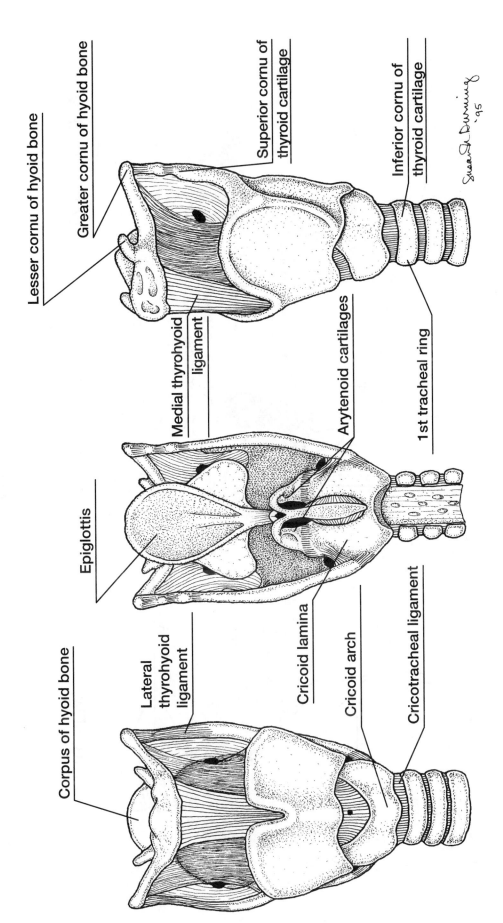

Lesser cornu of hyoid bone

Greater cornu of hyoid bone

Superior cornu of thyroid cartilage

Inferior cornu of thyroid cartilage

Medial thyrohyoid ligament

Arytenoid cartilages

1st tracheal ring

Epiglottis

Corpus of hyoid bone

Lateral thyrohyoid ligament

Cricoid lamina

Cricoid arch

Cricotracheal ligament

SKELETON OF THE LARYNX

275

Epilglottis

Hyoid bone

Thyroid cartilage

Transverse arytenoid muscle

Thyroid gland

Tracheal cartilages

Thyroid notch

Oblique arytenoid muscles

Thyroid lamina

Posterior cricoarytenoid muscle

Cricothyroid muscles

ANTERIOR VIEW

POSTERIOR VIEW

LATERAL VIEW

LARNYX

276

1.   Cranium

2.   Frontal; temporal; sphenoid; parietal; occipital

3.   Zygomatic

4.   Mandible

5.   Oral; nasal; pharyngeal

6.   (Two) orbits, the nasal cavity, and the cranial cavity

7.   The forehead (frons)

8.   Palatoglossus muscles

9.   Tongue; velum

10.   "Cleft palate"

11.   Orbicularis oris

12.   Oral stage

13.   Temporalis; masseter; and medial (internal) pterygoid muscles

14.   Velum; tongue; mandible

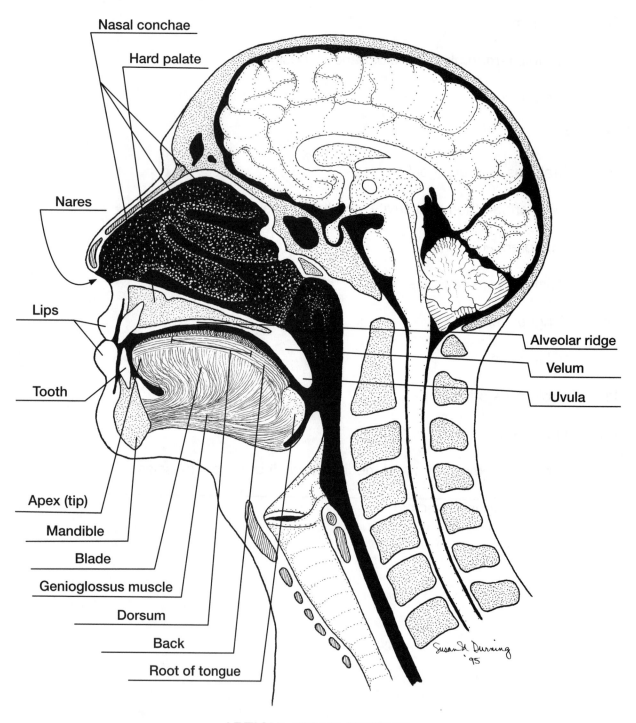

Nasal conchae

Hard palate

Nares

Lips

Tooth

Apex (tip)

Mandible

Blade

Genioglossus muscle

Dorsum

Back

Root of tongue

Alveolar ridge

Velum

Uvula

Susan St. Durning
'95

ARTICULATORY SYSTEM

278

Levator labii superioris muscle

Zygomaticus minor muscle

Zygomaticus major muscle

Orbicularis oris muscle

Levator anguli oris muscle

Risorius muscle

Depressor anguli oris muscle

Depressor labii inferioris muscle

MUSCLES OF FACIAL EXPRESSION

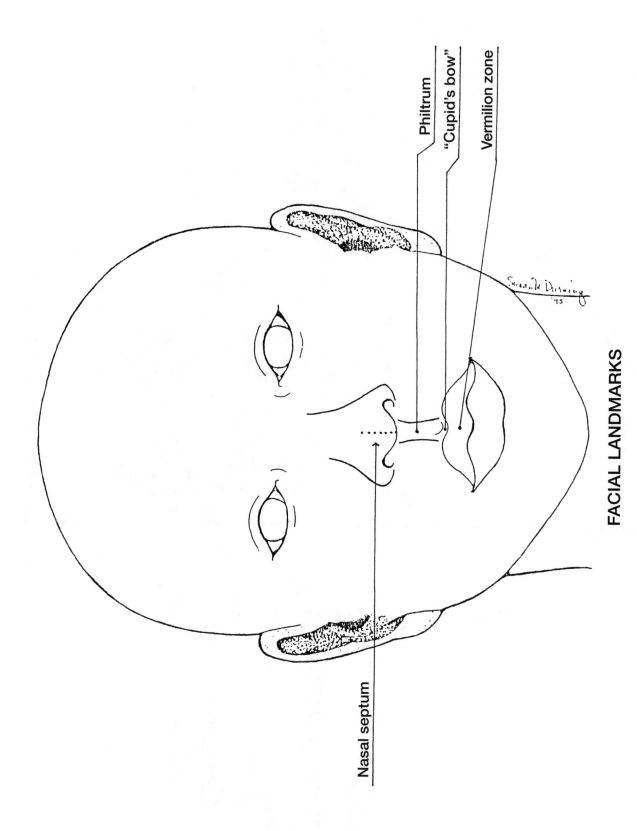

Philtrum

"Cupid's bow"

Vermilion zone

Nasal septum

FACIAL LANDMARKS

280

Temporalis muscle

Masseter muscle

TEMPORALIS AND MASSETER MUSCLES

1. Central nervous system and peripheral nervous system

2. The brain and the spinal cord

3. Afferent

4. Efferent

5. Frontal

6. 12

7. Peripheral

8. Spinal and cranial nerves and autonomic nervous system

9. Sympathetic nervous system

10. The association areas of the cerebral cortex

11. Synapses

12. Gyri

13. Lateral sulcus (fissure of Sylvius)

14. Central fissure (fissure of Rolando)

15. Sensory (tactile) reception

16. Pars triangularis of the left frontal lobe

17. Homonymous hemianopsia

18. Paralysis of the contralateral musculature

19. Brainstem

20. Hypoglossal nerve (XII).

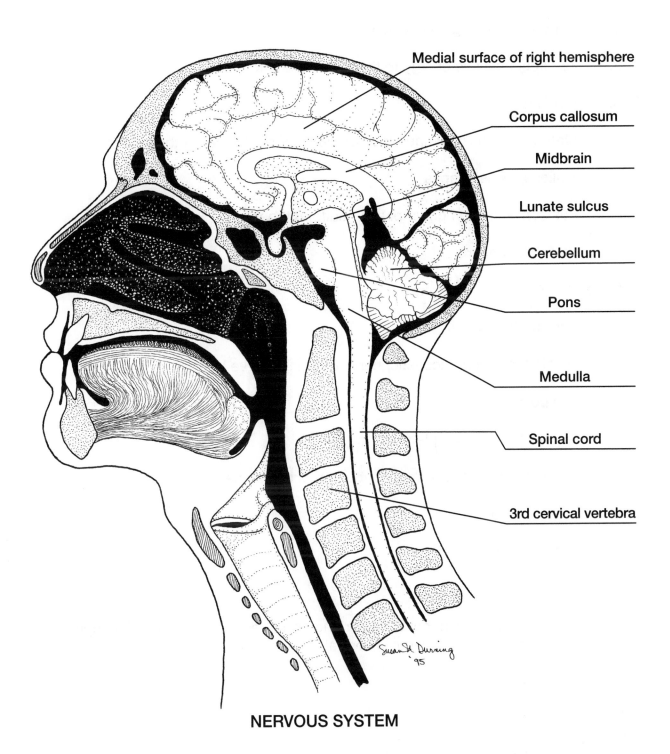

Medial surface of right hemisphere

Corpus callosum

Midbrain

Lunate sulcus

Cerebellum

Pons

Medulla

Spinal cord

3rd cervical vertebra

NERVOUS SYSTEM

1. Peripheral hearing mechanism

2. To direct acoustic energy to the external auditory meatus.

3. Cartilage

4. Match the acoustic impedance of the inner ear to that of the environment.

5. Malleus; incus; stapes

6. Eustachian (pharyngotympanic; auditory) tubes

7. Vestibular apparatus

8. Cochlea

9. Perilymph

10. Vestibulocochlear (acoustic) nerve or cranial nerve VIII

11. The pons

12. Superior olivary complex

13. Cerebral cortex of the dominant cerebral hemisphere

14. Temporal lobe

15. Cochlear nuclei

16. Acoustic neuroma

17. a) peripheral; b) peripheral; c) peripheral; d) central; e) central; f) peripheral;
    g) peripheral; h) peripheral; i) central; j) peripheral

18. Vestibular

19. Malleus

20. External ear, middle ear, and inner ear

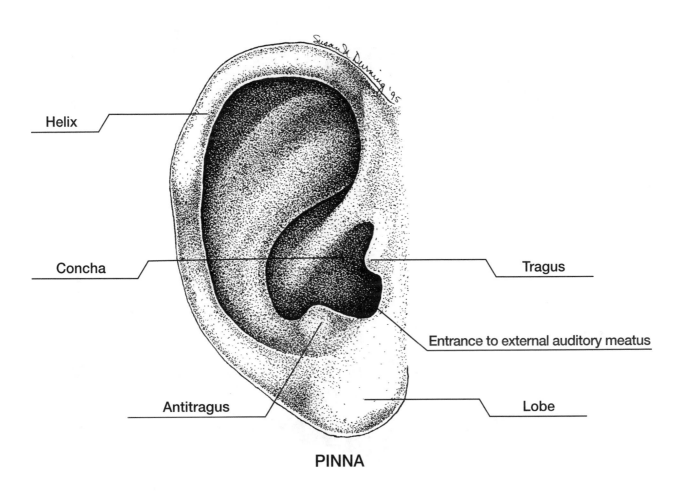

Helix

Concha

Tragus

Entrance to external auditory meatus

Antitragus

Lobe

PINNA

285

Semicircular canals

Cochlea

External auditory meatus

Auditory nerve

Stapes

Incus

Malleus

Tympanic membrane

Pinna

Stapedius muscle

Susan L. Durning
'95

CORONAL VIEW OF PERIPHERAL HEARING MECHANISM

INDEX